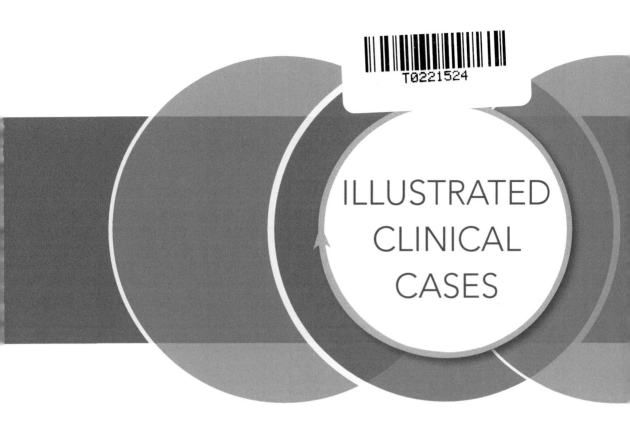

T0221524

# ILLUSTRATED CLINICAL CASES

# Cardiac Imaging

## SHAHID HUSSAIN
MA MB BChir MRCP FRCR
Consultant Cardiothoracic Radiologist
Heart of England NHS Foundation Trust, Birmingham, UK

## JONATHAN PANTING
BSc MB BChir FRCP
Consultant Cardiologist
Heart of England NHS Foundation Trust, Birmingham, UK

## JUN KIAT TEOH
MB ChB (Hons) (Edin) MRCP
Specialist Regsitrar in Cardiology
University Hospital Birmingham, Birmingham, UK

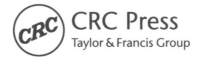

CRC Press
Taylor & Francis Group

CRC Press
Taylor & Francis Group
6000 Broken Sound Parkway NW, Suite 300
Boca Raton, FL 33487-2742

© 2014 by Taylor & Francis Group, LLC
CRC Press is an imprint of Taylor & Francis Group, an Informa business

No claim to original U.S. Government works

Printed on acid-free paper
Version Date: 20140121

International Standard Book Number-13: 978-1-4822-3573-9 (Paperback)

This book contains information obtained from authentic and highly regarded sources. While all reasonable efforts have been made to publish reliable data and information, neither the author[s] nor the publisher can accept any legal responsibility or liability for any errors or omissions that may be made. The publishers wish to make clear that any views or opinions expressed in this book by individual editors, authors or contributors are personal to them and do not necessarily reflect the views/opinions of the publishers. The information or guidance contained in this book is intended for use by medical, scientific or health-care professionals and is provided strictly as a supplement to the medical or other professional's own judgement, their knowledge of the patient's medical history, relevant manufacturer's instructions and the appropriate best practice guidelines. Because of the rapid advances in medical science, any information or advice on dosages, procedures or diagnoses should be independently verified. The reader is strongly urged to consult the drug companies' printed instructions, and their websites, before administering any of the drugs recommended in this book. This book does not indicate whether a particular treatment is appropriate or suitable for a particular individual. Ultimately it is the sole responsibility of the medical professional to make his or her own professional judgements, so as to advise and treat patients appropriately. The authors and publishers have also attempted to trace the copyright holders of all material reproduced in this publication and apologize to copyright holders if permission to publish in this form has not been obtained. If any copyright material has not been acknowledged please write and let us know so we may rectify in any future reprint.

---

**Library of Congress Cataloging-in-Publication Data**

---

Cardiac imaging (Hussain)
   Cardiac imaging / editors, Shahid Hussain, Jonathan Panting, Jun Kiat Teoh.
   p. ; cm. -- (Illustrated clinical cases)
   Includes bibliographical references and index.
   ISBN 978-1-4822-3573-9 (pbk. : alk. paper)
   I. Hussain, Shahid M., editor. II. Panting, Jonathan, editor. III. Teoh, Jun Kiat, editor. IV. Title. V. Series: Illustrated clinical cases.
   [DNLM: 1. Cardiovascular Diseases--diagnosis--Case Reports. 2. Cardiac Imaging Techniques--methods--Case Reports. WG 141]

RC670
616.1'2075--dc23                    2014001311

---

**Visit the Taylor & Francis Web site at**
**http://www.taylorandfrancis.com**

**and the CRC Press Web site at**
**http://www.crcpress.com**

# CONTENTS

# DEDICATION

Thank you to my family, for their love and support – SH

Thanks to Kim, Jack and Lottie for their patience – JP

I am forever indebted to my parents for their unwavering support, selfless sacrifice and above all else, for their unconditional love – JKT

# PREFACE

Cardiac imaging can take a multitude of forms. The basic chest radiograph can be the first identifier of cardiac disease, while dynamic imaging with echocardiography can provide immediate information about cardiac structure and function. Cross-sectional imaging in the form of computed tomography (CT) and cardiac magnetic resonance imaging (MRI) can provide information about cardiac structure and abnormalities, and MRI is frequently used to assess cardiac viability. Both techniques can be used in the diagnosis and assessment of congenital heart disease. Coronary artery imaging can be performed with invasive angiography and cardiac CT – with invasive angiography having the added dimension of intravascular ultrasound and the opportunity for intervention. Stress echocardiography; perfusion MRI; nuclear medicine myocardial perfusion (MIBI) scans and the emerging stress cardiac CT can provide information about the inducibility of cardiac ischaemia in patients with coronary artery disease. There are clearly many modalities which are used to image the heart and this variety and number of scan types can prove daunting to radiologists and cardiologists. In addition, there are the numerous devices, stents, valves and other paraphernalia which are employed in the management of cardiac disease, which need to be recognised and identified when interpreting any of these various scans.

We have attempted in this short book to present a variety of the common and not so common cardiac pathologies with imaging modalities which cover the spectrum of cardiac imaging. Thorough details about pathology, as well as the background of the imaging modality, are included in the discussion of each case. Hopefully it will encourage further reading and will prove useful to cardiologists/radiologists preparing for specialist examinations.

# ACKNOWLEDGEMENTS

The authors would like to acknowledge the invaluable contributions of

- Dr Debbie Wai, FRCR – Consultant Radiologist, Ealing Hospital NHS Trust
- Dr Hefin Jones, MBBS, BSc, FRCR – Consultant Cardiothoracic Radiologist, University Hospital North Staffordshire NHS Trust
- Dr Vijaya Pakala, MRCS, FRCR – Specialist Registrar in Radiology, Heart of England NHS Foundation Trust

all of whom contributed by helping to write cases for the book.

We would also like to acknowledge the help of Dr Helen Alton and Dr Mini Pakkal both of whom kindly contributed images for the book.

# CLASSIFICATION OF CASES

Aorta, thoracic: 5, 13, 42, 50, 52

Arrhythmias: 21, 61, 73

Cardiomyopathy: 49, 66

Congenital/anatomical anomalies: 1, 7, 9, 10, 14, 22, 33, 34, 39, 57, 62, 63, 64, 67, 69, 74

Coronary artery disease: 2, 3, 18, 25, 32, 36, 40, 45, 70, 71

Heart failure: 8, 10, 19, 27, 48

Infective disorders: 20, 24, 48

Infiltrative heart disorders: 15, 38

Investigative procedures: 4, 32, 40, 45, 46, 73, 64, 68, 73, 75

Ischaemic heart disease: 3, 4, 11, 12, 18, 27, 35, 36, 45, 46, 56, 60, 70, 71

Left ventricle (LV) disease: 31, 47, 54, 56, 72, 73

Paediatric cases: 10, 33, 63

Pericardial disease: 17, 29, 41, 51

Pulmonary vascular disease: 30, 44

Therapeutic procedures: 12, 16, 23, 35, 55, 61, 70, 71

Thromboembolism: 21, 26, 30, 56, 64, 65, 73

Tumours: 29, 37, 44, 59

Valvular heart disease: 6, 16, 20, 26, 28, 43, 53, 58, 75

# LIST OF ABBREVIATIONS

| | |
|---|---|
| ACC | American College of Cardiology |
| AF | atrial fibrillation |
| AHA | American Heart Association |
| ASA | atrial septal aneurysm |
| ASD | atrioseptal defect |
| AV | aortic valve |
| AVA | aortic valve area |
| AVR | aortic valve replacement |
| CABG | coronary artery bypass graft |
| CAD | coronary artery disease |
| CCS | Canadian Cardiovascular Society |
| CK | creatine kinase |
| CMR | cardiac magnetic resonance imaging |
| CRP | C-reactive protein |
| CRT | cardiac resynchronisation therapy |
| CT | computed tomography |
| CTPA | computed tomography pulmonary angiography |
| CXR | chest x-ray |
| DES | drug-eluting stent |
| ECG | electrocardiogram |
| ESC | European Society of Cardiology |
| ESR | eythrocyte sedimentation rate |
| ETT | exercise tolerance test |
| GP | general practitioner |
| GTN | glyceryl trinitrate |
| HIV | human immunodeficiency virus |
| HOCM | hypertrophic cardiac myopathy |
| IABP | intra-aortic balloon pump |
| ICD | implantable cardioverter-defbrillator |
| IVC | inferior vena cava |
| IVUS | intravascular ultrasound |
| LA | left atrium |
| LAD | left anterior descending (artery) |
| LBBB | left bundle branch block |
| LCA | left coronary artery |
| LMS | left main stem |
| LV | left ventricle |
| LVEF | left ventricular ejection fraction |
| LVF | left ventricular failure |
| LVOT | left ventricular outflow tract |
| MAC | mitral annular calcification |
| MI | myocardial infarction |
| MIBI | 2-methoxy isobutyl isonitrile |
| MPI | myocardial perfusion imaging |
| MRI | magnetic resonance imaging |
| MVP | mitral valve prolapse |
| NICE | National Institute for Clinical Excellence |
| NT-proBNP | N-terminal pro-brain natriuretic peptide |
| NYHA | New York Heart Association |
| PA | pulmonary artery |
| PCI | percutaneous coronary intervention |
| PDA | patent ductus arteriosus |
| PE | pulmonary embolus |
| PET | positron emission tomography |
| PFO | patent foramen ovale |
| PTMC | percutaneous transvenous mitral commissurotomy |
| RA | right atrium |
| RBBB | right bundle branch block |
| RCA | right coronary artery |
| RV | right ventricle |
| RVOT | right ventricular outflow tract |
| SOB | shortness of breath |
| SPECT | single photon emission computed tomography |
| STEMI | ST elevation myocardial infarction |
| SVC | superior vena cava |
| TB | tuberculosis |
| TGA | transposition of great arteries |
| TIA | transient ischaemic attack |
| TIMI | thrombolysis in myocardial infarction |
| TOE | transoesophageal echocardiogram |
| TOF | tetralogy of Fallot |
| TR | tricuspid regurgitation |
| TTE | transthoracic echocardiogram |
| VSD | ventriculoseptal defect |
| VVI | ventricle paced, ventricle sensed; pacing inhibited if beat sensed |

# QUESTION 1

1 A 40-year-old male presents to an accident and emergency department with acute onset of chest pain that was brought on by heavy lifting. There was no past history of angina. He was a smoker of 10 cigarettes per day for 15 years but had no other risk factors for coronary artery disease. Clinical examination, cardiac enzymes, ECG and CXR were all normal. The pain was relieved by paracetamol analgesia and was thought to be musculoskeletal in origin. However, given the slight uncertainty and the smoking history an out-patient cardiac CT was organised (1a, b).

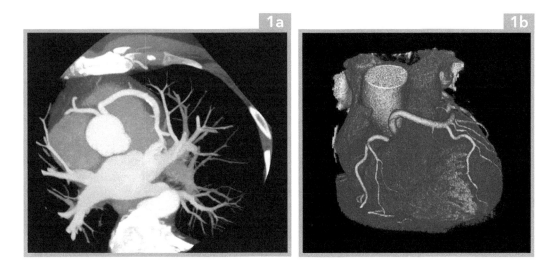

i. What does the cardiac CT demonstrate?

ii. What is the clinical significance of this abnormality?

## Answer 1

**1i.** The CT shows an aberrant LMS – nonmalignant.

The LMS normally arises from the left/posterior coronary sinus. In this case the LMS is arising from the anterior coronary sinus. It is usually 5–10 mm in length and does not vary in diameter. It passes posterior to the pulmonary trunk and bifurcates into 1) the LAD artery, which extends anteriorly in the interventricular groove to supply the septum and anterior wall of the LV; and 2) the circumflex artery which extends into the posterior arterioventricular groove to supply the lateral wall of the LV. The LMS can trifurcate to give a ramus intermedius branch which follows the course similar to that of a first diagonal branch of the LAD. In a left dominant system the circumflex gives rise to the posterior descending coronary artery.

The LCA arises from the right sinus of Valsalva as a separate vessel or as a branch of a single coronary artery in 0.09–0.11% of patients who undergo angiography. A malignant or interarterial course is associated with 75% of cases where the LMS arises from the right coronary sinus. These patients are at risk of sudden cardiac death as the vessel can become compressed between the aorta and the pulmonary artery, and because of the slit-like origin due to the acute angle that the vessel makes to pass posteriorly. The example shown, however, is of a prepulmonic course which is a nonmalignant course. The vessel has a widely patent origin and there is no risk of vascular compression; therefore, there is no risk of acute myocardial infarction.

**ii.** This is a nonmalignant course and is therefore simply an incidental finding.

# QUESTION 2

2 A 59-year-old male presents to hospital with severe crushing chest pain and profuse sweating while at work. He is a nonsmoker and denies any recreational drug use. His medication history includes ranitidine for heartburn and paracetamol for occasional migraine. His admission 12-lead ECG showed inferior ST elevation consistent with a clinical diagnosis of acute myocardial infarction. He was brought to the catheterisation laboratory for emergent coronary angiography with the view to coronary stenting.

i. What does Figure 2a show?

ii. Following acquisition of Figure 2a, intracoronary nitrates were administered. Figure 2b was then acquired 1 minute later. What does it show?

iii. What is the aetiology for this patient's presentation?

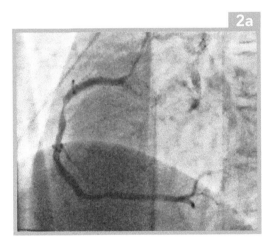 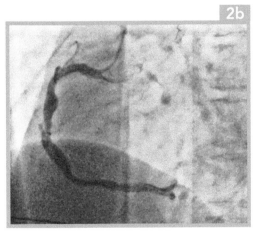

## Answer 2

**2i.** There is a severe discrete stenosis of the mid segment of the RCA (2c, arrow). In the context of the patient's presentation with crushing chest pain and inferior ECG changes, this is the culprit lesion.

**ii.** The overall diameter of the right coronary artery along its entire length has increased as a result of the vasodilatory effect of intracoronary nitrates. The discrete stenosis noted on Figure 2c (arrow) has now resolved, with no apparent stenosis seen on Figure 2d (arrow). No coronary stenting was required. The patient's symptoms and ECG changes resolved following nitrates administration.

**iii.** The cause of this patient's chest pain and ischaemic ECG changes is due to coronary vasospasm. Coronary vasospasm occurs due to smooth muscle constriction of coronary arteries. The exact pathophysiological mechanism of why some patients get significant vasospasm, occasionally leading to frank myocardial infarction, is not clearly understood. Commonly described triggers for coronary vasospasm in individuals who are susceptible include hyperventilation, cocaine or amphetamine use, cigarette smoking and exposure to cold. There is overall a slight female preponderance. The overall prognosis of this condition is generally good, although in affected patients there may be significant morbidity in the form of frequent chest pain which may have considerable impact on quality of life. In the CASPAR trial (Coronary Artery Spasm in Patients with Acute Coronary Syndrome), patients without culprit lesion and proven coronary vasospasm had an excellent prognosis. The pharmacological treatment for patients with coronary vasospasm to prevent recurrent spasms is calcium channel blocker and long-acting nitrates. Nonselective beta-blockers may worsen symptoms as blockade of the beta-receptors can result in unopposed alpha-receptor-mediated vasoconstriction to occur. It is not uncommon for patients with coronary vasospasm to be mistakenly diagnosed as having a *bona fide* acute myocardial infarction due to plaque rupture, resulting in unnecessary stenting. It is therefore prudent to administer nitrates when encountering a radiographically stenotic lesion to exclude vasospasm so as to avoid needless intervention.

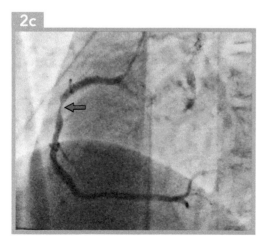

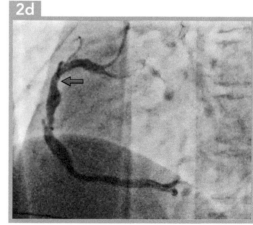

## QUESTION 3

3   A 65-year-old male is admitted with chest pain, a positive troponin and ST elevation on ECG. A CMR was requested (3a–c) to determine viability and whether the patient should go on to undergo invasive coronary angiography.

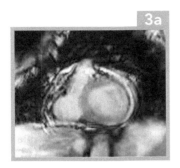
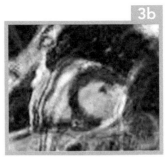

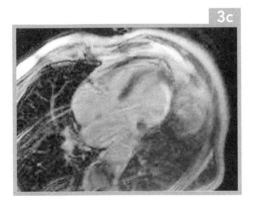

i.   What is the diagnosis?

ii.   Would this patient benefit from coronary revascularisation?

## Answer 3

**3i.** Figure 3a is a cine short-axis view at the base of the heart demonstrating significant myocardial wall thinning in the lateral wall. Figure 3b is an inversion recovery fast gradient-echo sequence with late gadolinium showing transmural late enhancement of the corresponding myocardial segments. Figure 3c is a four-chamber view with late gadolinium demonstrating transmural late enhancement in the lateral wall of the LV at the basal, mid and apical levels. The diagnosis is a circumflex territory infarct.

**ii.** The infarct in this case is considered to be nonviable. Hence the patient would not benefit from coronary revascularisation. An important and common application of CMR is the determination of myocardial viability. Only viable myocardial segments will benefit from coronary revascularisation and regain function, with improvements in ejection fraction and exercise capacity. Nonviable myocardium is scar tissue which has permanently lost its function. The detection of nonviable myocardium in patients with left ventricular dysfunction avoids patients undergoing invasive revascularisation procedures from which they are unlikely to benefit.

Dysfunctional but viable myocardium can be divided into two states – hibernating myocardium and stunned myocardium. Hibernating myocardium shows significant wall motion abnormality, but late enhancement is absent or limited. Stunned myocardium exhibits decreased contractile function, but does not show delayed enhancement. Stunned myocardium will recover spontaneously over time.

CMR is excellent at determining myocardial viability using late gadolinium. Traditionally, radionuclide myocardial perfusion imaging or stress echocardiography have been utilised to assess myocardial viability, but CMR is a technique which compares favourably to these modalities. The probability of improvement in segmental function significantly decreases as the extent of transmural late gadolinium enhancement increases. Less than 50% transmural enhancement has a high likelihood of functional recovery, while transmural infarction of 75% is unlikely to recover contractility. In addition, myocardial thinning (<5 mm) predicts nonviability. Regional wall motion abnormality does not serve alone to differentiate infarcted from hibernating myocardium. However, akinesia in the presence of transmural late gadolinium enhancement or wall thinning suggests nonviability.

# QUESTION 4

4  An 80-year-old female presents with a 6-month history of progressive shortness of breath while walking to the shops. She has never smoked but is overweight, diabetic and has hypertension. She has had no chest pain. She initially had a CT coronary artery calcium score assessment which demonstrated an agatston score of 895. She was not keen on an invasive test and therefore was referred for a functional test. She was only able to manage 2 minutes of an exercise tolerance test due to arthritis in her knees and was therefore referred for a MIBI scan (4).

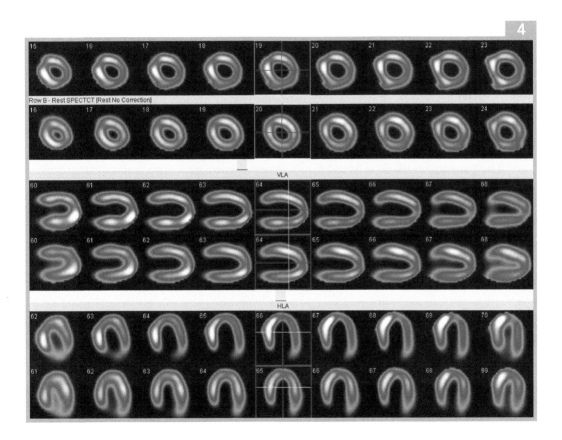

i.   What does the MIBI scan show?

ii.  What should the next investigation be?

## Answer 4

**4i.** The MIBI scan has some fairly subtle findings but is clearly abnormal. There is a defect in the lateral LV wall which can only really be appreciated on the horizontal long-axis images. There is poor uptake of isotope on the stress images, with a reversible defect demonstrated since there is relatively normal uptake on the rest images. This would be consistent with reversible ischaemia in the circumflex artery territory.

Calcium scoring is a useful tool in identifying risk of a coronary event in patients. A test is considered to be positive if calcification is detected within the coronary arteries – and the amount of calcification is quantified using the agatston scoring system. Absolute agatston scores of <10, 11–99, 100–400, and >400 have been proposed to categorise individuals into groups having minimal, moderate, significant, or extensive amounts of calcification, respectively. Patients with a score of >400 have been shown to have a higher risk of myocardial events and a higher incidence of interventions – angioplasty/CABG. In elderly patients (>70 years) patients with a score of >400 have a higher risk of death.

**ii.** The patient should be referred for an invasive angiogram. The scan has suggested reversible ischaemia in a single vessel and the patient would potentially be a candidate for angioplasty +/- stent.

# QUESTION 5

5 A 76-year-old female is woken up in the middle of the night with upper back pain in between her shoulder blades. Her son brought her to the emergency department in some distress. The patient has a history of hypertension but was otherwise physically well. On examination, her heart sounds were pure with no murmurs. Her 12-lead ECG did not show any significant abnormalities. Her CXR showed some mediastinal widening. Her blood pressure measured on the left arm was 118/65 mmHg and on the right 151/77 mmHg. The cardiology registrar was requested to perform an urgent transthoracic echocardiogram (5a, b).

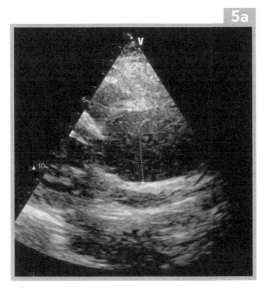
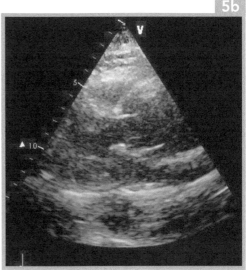

i. What do the echocardiographic images show?

ii. What is the immediate management for this patient?

iii. What conditions are associated with aortic dissection?

iv. What is the prognosis of aortic dissection?

**5i.** The echocardiographic images show a dilated aortic root in the parasternal long-axis view (5a). Following a slight tilt of the ultrasound probe, a dissection flap can be seen (5c, arrow) within the aortic root. The diagnosis for this patient is acute aortic dissection on a background of an aneurysmal aortic root.

**ii.** The immediate priority is to stabilise the patient while confirming the diagnosis and extent of the dissection. Blood pressure control is imperative in patients who have confirmed aortic dissection, with the aim of achieving systolic blood pressure of between 100 mmHg and 120 mmHg. In the absence of contraindications, intravenous beta-blockers (e.g. labetalol) are recommended as first-line agents. If additional antihypertensives are required, vasodilators such as intravenous nitrates or sodium nitroprusside can be used. The general rule is that patients with involvement of the ascending aorta should have emergency surgical repair. Surgery is also indicated if there is evidence of rupture (e.g. into the pericardial space causing haemopericardium), arterial compromise (e.g. limb ischaemia, renal perfusion compromise) or progression of dissection on serial imaging and with ongoing pain.

**iii.** Uncontrolled hypertension, connective tissue disorders (Marfan's syndrome, Ehlers–Danlos syndrome), vascular inflammation (giant cell arteritis, Takayasu's arteritis), deceleration trauma (motor vehicle accident) and iatrogenic causes (cardiac catheterisation) are associated with aortic dissection.

**iv.** Acute aortic dissection is associated with a high mortality rate. The mortality for untreated aortic dissection is about 20–30% at 24 hours and about 65–70% at 2 weeks. Operative mortality is between 10% and 25% and is linked to a significant extent to the patient's premorbid general health.

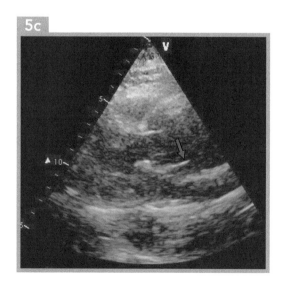

## QUESTION 6

6 A 50-year-old male presents with dyspnoea on exertion, orthopnoea and paroxysmal nocturnal dyspnoea. He also complains of palpitations. On examination, a diastolic murmur could be heard.

i. What are the image findings and diagnosis (6a, b)?

ii. Describe the standard MR techniques for quantitative evaluation.

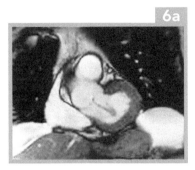

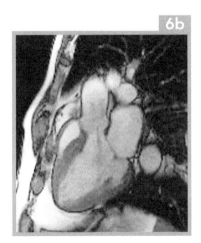

## Answer 6

**6i.** Figure 6a is a cine gradient–echo sequence of the left ventricular outflow tract. Figure 6b is a cine three-chamber view. A signal void jet arising from the aortic valve is demonstrated in both images consistent with aortic regurgitation.

Aortic regurgitation can be due to leaflet abnormalities resulting from infective endocarditis and rheumatic heart disease. It can also be due to aortic root dilatation (annuloaortic ectasia) which may be idiopathic, age related or secondary to, for example, hypertension, aortitis and Marfan's syndrome. A bicuspid valve may lead to aortic regurgitation. Aortic regurgitation can also be due to dissection, trauma and aneurysm.

Aortic regurgitation results in volume overload of the LV. Ventricular dilatation and increased LV compliance are compensatory mechanisms that allow increased stroke volume and preservation of cardiac output. However, when LV function begins to deteriorate, both end-systolic and end-diastolic volumes increase. This can be quantified with cine MRI along with stroke volume and ejection fraction.

Patients with aortic regurgitation are closely monitored for LV dysfunction as they may require surgery even while asymptomatic, before irreversible LV dysfunction occurs. MRI can be used to evaluate ventricular function, and help in determining when surgical intervention is indicated.

**ii.** Quantitative information regarding the severity of regurgitant lesions can be obtained by using a combination of cine gradient-echo or steady-state free precession and cine phase contrast sequences.

Phase contrast imaging uses bipolar gradients to produce phase changes in moving blood. The phase change is related to the flow velocity. Time–velocity and time–flow curves can be generated by drawing a region of interest around a vessel or flow jet of interest. In the case of aortic regurgitation, the imaging plane is performed perpendicular to the AV positioned just above the valve. If a time–flow graph is plotted, the area under the curve below zero is equal to the regurgitant volume.

Cine MR allows an alternative method for quantifying the degree of aortic regurgitation by ventricular volumetric measurements. The difference between the stroke volumes of the LV and RV is equal to the regurgitant volume. The regurgitant fraction is the regurgitant volume divided by the total stroke volume. This is assuming that there is no intracardiac shunt and that the other valves are competent.

## QUESTION 7

7    An 18-year-old male attends accident and emergency following an injury to his chest playing rugby. He complains of chest pain and a CXR was requested as part of his investigations (7a).

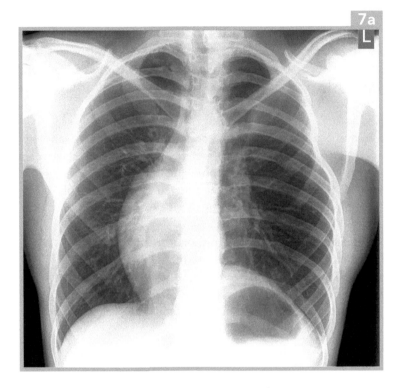

i.    What is the diagnosis?

ii.   List some other causes of unilateral hyperlucent hemithorax.

## Answer 7

**7i.** The CXR shows dextrocardia and hyperlucency of the left hemithorax, relative to the right. There is also absence of the left pectoralis major muscle shadow. Physical examination revealed webbing of the digits of the left hand. The patient incidentally has Poland syndrome. The CT thorax demonstrates these findings more clearly, in particular absence of the left pectoralis major (7b).

Poland syndrome was first described by Alfred Poland, an English surgeon, in 1841. It is characterised by unilateral absence/partial absence of the sternocostal head of the pectoralis major muscle (commonly) or pectoralis minor, ipsilateral syndactyly and brachydactyly, rib anomalies and aplasia of the breast or nipple. There is an association with dextrocardia.

Poland syndrome is a rare congenital condition, of unknown aetiology, but the theory is that it is due to interruption of the embryonic subclavian and vertebral arteries in early gestation. The syndrome affects males more than females with a ratio of 3:1. The right hemithorax is affected more commonly than the left. Patients may undergo cosmetic reconstructive surgery.

**ii.** Causes of unilateral hyperlucent hemithorax include:
- Technical factors: rotation of the patient.
- Chest wall abnormality: mastectomy, scoliosis.
- Airways disease: pneumothorax, emphysema.
- Vascular disease: pulmonary embolism, pulmonary artery obstruction, pulmonary artery hypoplasia.

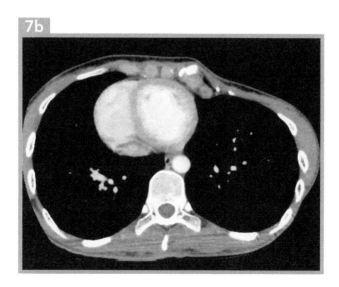

7b

## QUESTION 8

8   A 75-year-old male is referred by his GP to the heart failure clinic because of
a 6-month history of worsening breathlessness, orthopnoea and peripheral leg
swelling. The patient had an anterior myocardial infarction 11 years ago and his
last echocardiogram, performed 5 years ago prior to an elective hip replacement,
showed mild left ventricular systolic dysfunction. His NT-proBNP level measured
by his GP was 1680 pg/ml. His clinical examination revealed evidence of
congestive heart failure and overall he is in NYHA class III. An up-to-date
transthoracic echocardiogram confirmed severe left ventricular systolic dysfunction
with an ejection fraction of 23%, with an akinetic anterior wall and a dyskinetic
septum. His 12-lead ECG showed that he is in sinus rhythm at a rate of 68 bpm
with a LBBB pattern (QRS duration 158 ms). He was referred for CRT.

i.   The CXR shown was performed after the patient had his CRT. What do the
arrows point to in Figure 8a?

ii.  What is CRT?

iii. What are the criteria in selecting patients for CRT?

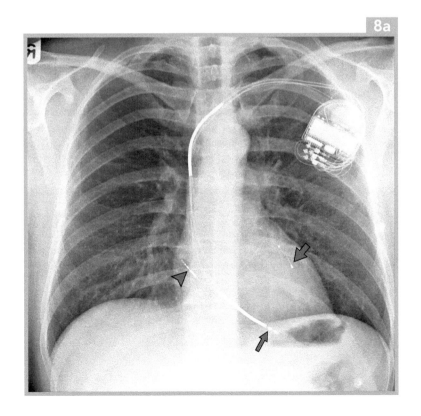

**8i.** The arrowhead points to the right atrial lead which is positioned in the right atrial appendage. The large arrow points to the left ventricular lead and it is positioned within a cardiac vein (this is manoeuvred into position via the coronary sinus). The small arrow is pointing towards the right ventricular lead and in this patient this is also the defibrillator lead. The corresponding leads are shown in the lateral x-ray projection (8b).

**ii.** Compared to patients with normal heart function who have a narrow QRS width, patients with severe systolic dysfunction often have conduction delay seen as a wide QRS duration (usually a LBBB) which is associated with mechanical dyssynchrony. Cardiac dyssynchrony results in a decrease in stroke volume and ejection fraction. CRT, also known as biventricular pacing, involves near-simultaneous pacing of both the left and right ventricle, with the overall aim of improving/restoring ventricular synchrony in these patients. A significant proportion of patients who are eligible for CRT will also fulfill indications for an implantable cardioverter-defibrillator. If this is the case then the patient should be considered for a CRT-D device (as opposed to a CRT-P device).

**iii.** The ESC has given a Class I recommendation for CRT-P or D to reduce morbidity and mortality in patients who meet the following criteria: NYHA class III/IV symptoms (class IV patients should be ambulatory); LVEF ≤35%; QRS ≥120 ms; in sinus rhythm; and on optimal medical therapy. In patients with NYHA Class III/IV heart failure who meet the criteria for CRT, multiple randomised control trials have demonstrated a significant benefit in terms of symptoms and an increase in exercise capacity. The 6 minute walk distance is increased by an average of 20%, with a resultant improvement in quality of life. CRT has also been shown to reduce the rate of hospitalisation for heart failure. In the landmark CARE-HF trial, where CRT-P was assessed, there was a statistically significant 36% relative risk reduction in mortality after a mean follow up of 29 months. There is also evidence to support some degree of reverse remodelling with CRT, with reductions in left ventricular end-diastolic diameter and improvement in LVEF.

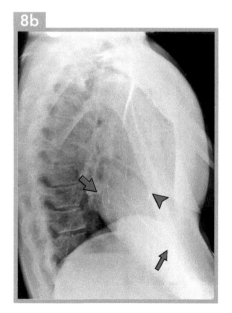

8b

## QUESTION 9

**9** A 25-year-old professional football player with a strong family history of coronary artery disease presents to his GP with a history of exercise-related chest pain. There is a smoking history of 3–4 cigarettes per day for 10 years. No other risk factors are identified. Clinical examination, cardiac enzymes, ECG and CXR were all completely normal.

**i.** What does the cardiac CT show (9a, b)?

**ii.** How frequently is this abnormality seen and what is its clinical importance?

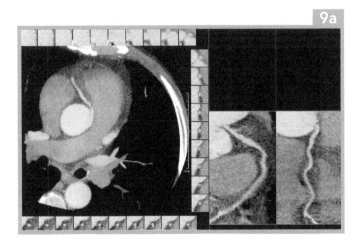

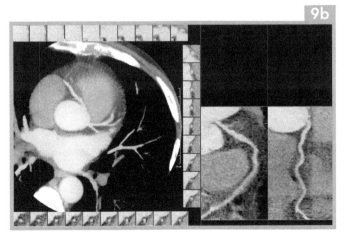

**9i.** CT shows an aberrant RCA with a malignant course.

The RCA arises from the anterior or right coronary sinus and is usually at a level which is inferior to the corresponding origin of the left main stem. The RCA passes to the right of the pulmonary artery and then descends in the anterior atrioventricular groove towards the posterior interventricular septum. The RCA branches consist of firstly the conus artery; then the sinoatrial nodal branch; then at the junction between the mid and distal RCA is the acute marginal branch. In 70% of cases the RCA is the dominant vessel and gives off the posterior descending artery and a posterolateral branch.

The RCA arises from the left sinus of Valsalva as a separate vessel or as a branch of a single coronary artery in 0.03–0.17% of patients who undergo angiography. The commonest course is interarterial, as shown here. This course can be associated with sudden cardiac death in up to 30% of patients. The pathophysiology is believed to be that during exercise, when there is slight dilatation of the aorta, the slit-like origin of the RCA becomes compressed between the aorta and pulmonary artery, resulting in ischaemia that may in severe cases lead to myocardial infarction. This path is termed a malignant course.

**ii.** Coronary artery anomalies are uncommon, with a reported prevalence ranging from 0.2% to 1.6%. Coronary anomalies can be fatal (typically in young, previously healthy athletes). In individuals aged between 14 and 40 years, coronary anomalies are involved in 12% of sports-related sudden cardiac deaths versus 1.2% of nonsports–related deaths.

## QUESTION 10

10 An MRI was performed on a neonate who developed congestive cardiac failure (10).

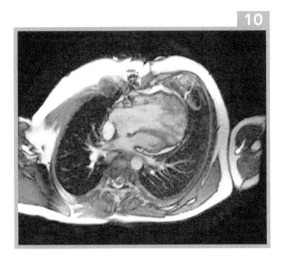

i.   What is the diagnosis?

ii.  How do these patients typically present?

iii. What are the treatment options?

## Answer 10

**10i.** The single axial MRI image demonstrates marked asymmetry between the LA/LV and the RA/RV with marked hypoplasia of the left. Appearances would be of a hypoplastic left heart syndrome.

Hypoplastic left heart syndrome, also called Shone syndrome, is a complex anomaly characterised by hypoplasia of the LA, LV, mitral/aortic valves and aorta. The incidence is 1 in 10,000 births with a male predilection. This represents 2–4% of congenital cardiac anomalies. Due to an underdeveloped LA and LV there is obstruction to the LVOT, so oxygenated blood from pulmonary veins passes into the RA through the foramen ovale. This causes increased load on the right heart and causes dilatation of the right heart and pulmonary arteries. Systemic perfusion occurs through a PDA. Survival requires a large PDA and ASD.

**ii.** Usually asymptomatic at birth, symptoms start after the closure of PDA. Common presentation is with heart failure, pulmonary hypertension, cardiogenic shock and cyanosis. This is one of the common causes of neonatal congestive cardiac failure and the fourth commonest cardiac anomaly in the first year of life. If untreated the condition can be fatal. Associations include aortic coarctation and endocardial fibroelastosis.

On CXR there can be a small, normal or enlarged cardiac silhouette. There can be features of pulmonary venous congestion. Echo demonstrates a hypoplastic ascending aorta; small but thick walled LV; the right heart chambers may be enlarged; and there may be impaired mitral valve movement. CT and MRI allow direct visualisation of anomaly and vessel anatomy.

**iii.** Treatment includes:
- Prostaglandin E to keep the PDA patent +/–balloon dilatation of the ASD (Rashkind atrioseptostomy).
- Palliative Norwood procedure (PA and descending aorta conduit followed by PA banding).
- Fontan procedure (RA connected directly to the PA).
- Heart transplant.

20

# QUESTION 11

11 A 60-year-old male presents with typical angina chest pain. He is hypertensive, diabetic and has a family history of ischaemic heart disease. A radionuclide perfusion study was inconclusive and so a stress perfusion MRI was requested (11a–d). Figure 11a is the adenosine stress perfusion image, 11b is the rest perfusion image and 11c, d are with late gadolinium.

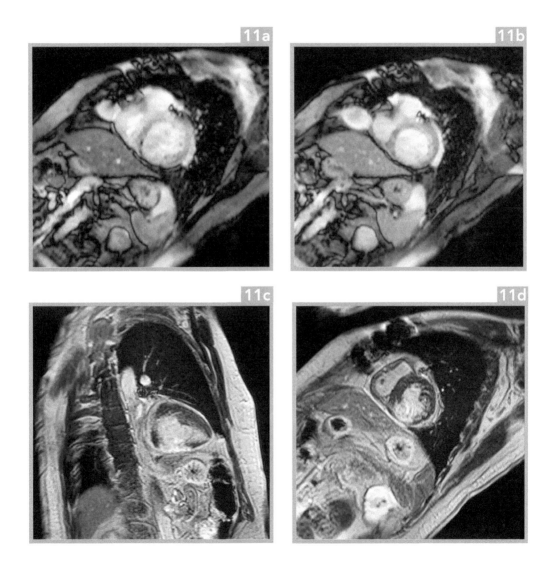

i.     What are the MRI findings?

ii.     According to the AHA, how many segments can the LV be divided into?

## Answer 11

**11i.** The adenosine stress perfusion image shows hypoenhancement in the inferoseptal walls at the mid LV level. The rest perfusion image shows normal enhancement of the myocardium in the inferoseptal segment but thinning in the inferior segment. The two-chamber late gadolinium image (11c) shows transmural late enhancement in the basal and mid LV level inferior wall. This is confirmed on the late gadolinium short-axis image (11d). The findings indicate reversible ischaemia in the inferoseptal wall. The patient would benefit from coronary revascularisation. There is also an infarct in the inferior wall – right coronary artery territory, considered nonviable.

**ii.** According to the AHA, the LV can be named and divided into 17 segments for the purposes of regional wall motion abnormality or myocardial perfusion (11e). In this model, the LV is divided into thirds perpendicular to the long axis of the heart, giving rise to basal, mid and apical levels:

- The basal level is divided into six segments: *basal anterior, anteroseptal, inferoseptal, inferior, inferolateral* and *anterolateral*.
- The mid level is divided into six segments: *mid anterior, anteroseptal, inferoseptal, inferior, inferolateral* and *anterolateral*.
- The apex is divided into four segments: *apical anterior, septal, inferior* and *lateral*.
- The apical cap contributes to one segment.

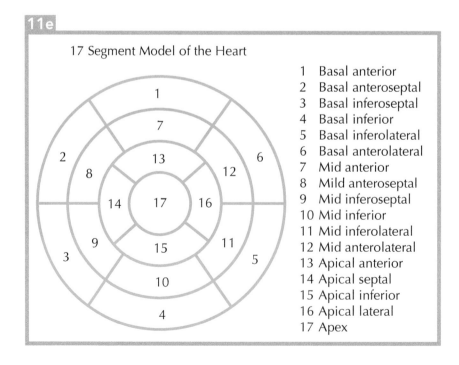

**11e**

17 Segment Model of the Heart

1 Basal anterior
2 Basal anteroseptal
3 Basal inferoseptal
4 Basal inferior
5 Basal inferolateral
6 Basal anterolateral
7 Mid anterior
8 Mild anteroseptal
9 Mid inferoseptal
10 Mid inferior
11 Mid inferolateral
12 Mid anterolateral
13 Apical anterior
14 Apical septal
15 Apical inferior
16 Apical lateral
17 Apex

12  A 65-year-old female presents to hospital with a 2-hour history of central chest pain which was confirmed to be an ST elevation myocardial infarction on arrival. She was emergently brought to the cardiac catheterisation laboratory for primary percutaneous coronary intervention. Her left anterior descending artery was found to be acutely occluded and this was dealt with by thrombus aspiration and coronary stenting. There was also moderate coronary artery disease in the right coronary artery. At the end of the procedure, the patient was hypotensive with a blood pressure of 82/45 mmHg. A decision was made to insert an IABP. A postprocedure CXR was performed (12).

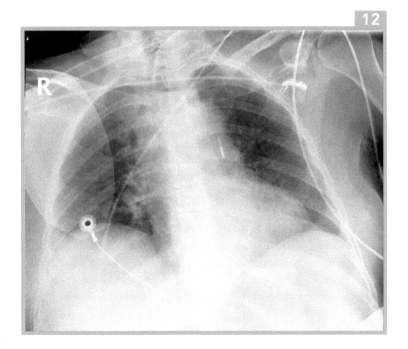

i.    What does the CXR show?

ii.   What is the role of an IABP?

iii.  What are the contraindications to having an IABP?

iv.   What are the potential complications?

## Answer 12

**12i.** Figure 12 is a portable CXR performed in the supine position because the patient has an IABP *in situ* which has been inserted via the left femoral artery. She is unable to sit up as it would impede the functioning of the IABP. A chest radiograph is mandatory after IABP insertion to check the position of the balloon tip. The radio-opaque tip of the IABP should lie between the second and third intercostal space to avoid occluding the left subclavian artery proximally and the renal arteries distally.

**ii.** International guidelines recommend the use of IABP counterpulsation as a Class I indication for patients with cardiogenic shock complicating acute MI. This view however, has been challenged more recently with the publication of the IABP-SHOCK II trial results which showed no reduction in 30-day mortality compared with controls. Other indications for IABP use are in patients with acute mitral regurgitation, VSD complicating MI and intractable ventricular arrhythmia due to myocardial ischaemia (as a bridge to definitive revascularisation). IABP is a temporary circulatory assist device which works on the principle of cardiac counter-pulsation. The balloon measures about 25 cm and is mounted on a catheter which is inserted via the femoral artery. The balloon, positioned within the descending aorta, is inflated during diastole and deflated during systole. The balloon inflation during diastole increases the coronary blood flow while the deflation in systole reduces left ventricular afterload and hence reduces myocardial work and oxygen consumption.

**iii.** An IABP is contraindicated in patients with severe aortic regurgitation and aortic dissection. Relative contraindications include bilateral ileofemoral disease, thoracic or abdominal aortic aneurysm and presence of severe coagulopathy.

**iv.** Limb ischaemia, aortic dissection, balloon rupture with air embolisation, septicaemia, stroke, access site vascular injury and acute kidney injury (from inadvertent renal artery occlusion by the balloon) are potential complications from IABP.

## QUESTION 13

13  A 64-year-old male with a history of hypercholesterolaemia and hypertension presents with acute onset of atypical chest pain and shortness of breath. He has smoked five cigarettes per day on and off for a period of ~20 years. His father had died of a heart attack at the age of 73 years and his 66-year-old brother had angina. He had never had any previous chest pain episodes. He is relatively fit and mobile with no other significant past medical history. The CXR was not of particularly good quality but showed a slightly widened mediastinum. Initial ECG was normal as was the troponin I. D-dimers were not raised. There was significant uncertainty about the underlying diagnosis but he continued to have significant chest pain which could not be controlled with glyceryl trinitrate/opiates and therefore a triple rule-out CT was performed (13a–d).

i.  What is the diagnosis?

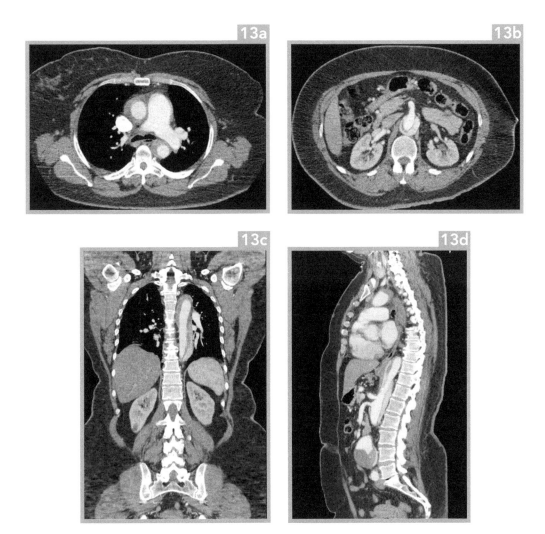

## Answer 13

**13i.** Figure 13a is an axial image through the chest and upper abdomen with contrast well opacifying the aorta. It demonstrates circumferential high attenuation material around the patent lumen of the aorta and appearances would be consistent with intramural haematoma. It is particularly useful in these patients initially to image with an uncontrasted scan of the chest since intramural blood is high attenuation on these images. Figure 13b demonstrates that the acute aortic pathology has progressed to a complete dissection with a spiralling luminal tear extending to involve the rest of the aorta.

Figure 13c is a coronal reformat and Figure 13d is a sagittal reformatted image of the entire aorta. They nicely demonstrate the two lumens of the aorta due to the dissection. The false lumen has a crescentic shape to it. It is also possible to identify a large 6.3 cm heavily thrombosed abdominal aortic aneurysm.

An aortic dissection occurs when blood splits the medial layer of the wall of the aorta. The aortic intima and adventitia become separated by blood. Aortic dissection can subsequently therefore lead to occlusion of branches of the aorta. Aortic dissection usually occurs by one of two underlying mechansisms. Most commonly (~95%) it can occur due to an aortic ulcer leading to a tear in the intima. Predisposing factors include cystic medial degeneration and hypertension. It can however, also occur due to primary haemorrhage into the aortic wall, with bleeding of the vasa vasorum causing intramural haematoma (~5% of cases).

Hypertension is the most significant underlying factor. Other predisposing risk factors include Marfan's syndrome, Ehlers–Danlos syndrome and pregnancy.

Aortic dissection can be classified using either the DeBakey or Stanford classifications. The Stanford classification system helps decide treatment. Usually, type A dissections require surgery, while type B dissections may be managed medically:
- Type A (60%) – dissection involves the ascending aorta and arch. This type of dissection is treated by emergency surgery. They can be complicated by rupture into the pericardium leading to caradiac tamponade, dissection of the coronary arteries and acute aortic valve insufficiency with acute heart failure.
- Type B (40%) – dissection involves the descending aorta only and begins after the left subclavian artery.

Management of intramural haematoma is the same as for that of an aortic dissection and therefore this patient would require emergency cardiothoracic vascular surgical referral for ascending aorta surgical repair.

# QUESTION 14

14  A 25-year-old male presents with worsening cyanosis, dyspnoea and had an abnormal ECG.

i.  What is the diagnosis (14)?

ii.  What are the imaging features?

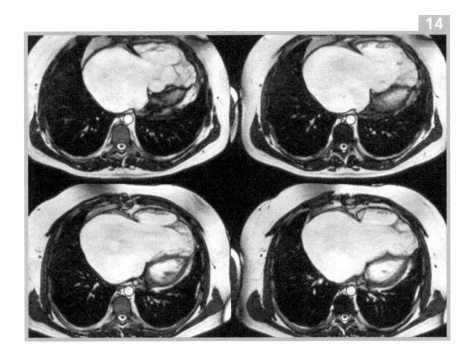

**14i.** The MRI images demonstrate a massive RA with a small atrialised portion of the RV and a small inferior chamber. Appearances would be consistent with Ebstein's anomaly.

**ii.** Ebstein's anomaly is a rare congenital cardiac abnormality occurring in fewer than 1 in 200,000 live births, where there is a large and fenestrated tricuspid valve with displacement of the tricuspid leaflets into the RV causing atrialisation of the superior RV. This is associated with trisomy 13, trisomy 21, Turner's syndrome, maternal lithium intake, PFO, ASD, VSD, pulmonary stenosis, mitral valve prolapse and coarctation of the aorta. There is an interatrial communication seen in ~90% of cases. There is RV hypoplasia with fibrosis, dilatation and secondary heart failure. Patients usually present with tricuspid regurgitation, atrioventricular re-entry tachycardia and arrhythmias. Prognosis is poor with 50% of patients dying in the first year of life.

There are various classification systems used for Ebstein's anomaly:
1. Carpentier classification:
   - Type A – the volume of the true RV is adequate.
   - Type B – large atrialised part of the RV, but the anterior leaflet of the tricuspid valve moves freely.
   - Type C – the anterior leaflet is significantly restricted and can cause RVOT obstruction.
   - Type D – almost complete atrialisation of the ventricle except for a small infundibular component.
2. Celermajer describes an echocardiographic grading system from 1 to 4 for neonates dependent on the ratio of RA/atrialised RV to functional RV.
3. On a plain chest radiograph the appearance can be of a box-shaped heart with horizontal position of the RVOT and right atrial enlargement. Echocardiography demonstrates apical displacement of the tricuspid valve by more than 8 mm/m$^2$ body surface area and an elongated anterior valve leaflet. It will also demonstrate a large RA with a small atrialised RV.

Usual presentation is at birth with cyanosis and symptoms of heart failure, dyspnoea, fatigue, supraventricular arrhythmias (Wolff–Parkinson–White syndrome), syncopal attacks, hepatomegaly and RBBB. There is usually a right-to-left shunt and the degree of cyanosis will depend upon the degree of pulmonary artery pressure.

Treatment includes:
- Prostaglandin therapy to keep the PDA open.
- Medical management of heart failure.
- Endocarditis prophylaxis.
- Arrhythmia control – antiarrhythmics/ablation/Maze procedure.
- Surgical correction of underlying tricuspid valve (repair/replacement) and RV abnormalities.

# QUESTION 15

15 A 34-year-old south Asian male had a chest radiograph in the emergency department following a fall. The CXR was abnormal and on further discussion it was discovered that the patient had symptoms of shortness of breath and a dry cough. He also reported a long-standing mild fever and some weight loss. He was referred back to his GP for further investigation.

**i.** What is the abnormality on these MR images (15a–c) and findings on CT lung windows (15d, e)?

**ii.** What are the common and associated pulmonary manifestations of this condition?

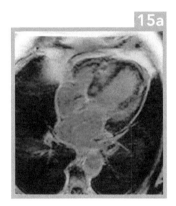

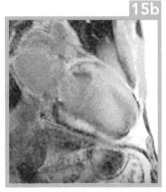

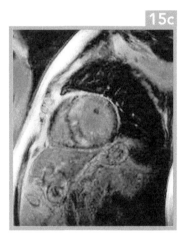

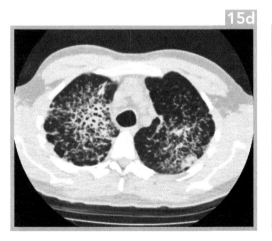

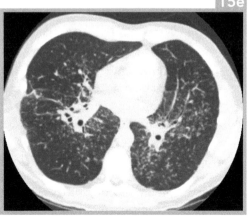

## Answer 15

**15i.** The MR images are from the late gadolinium stage of the investigation; four-chamber (15a), two-chamber (15b) and short-axis (15c) images are presented here. They show mild myocardial thickening and delayed intramural enhancement. These appearances would be consistent with an infiltrative nonischaemic disorder. The common conditions to give this distribution of late gadolinium enhancement include sarcoidosis, myocarditis, Fabry's disease and Chagas disease.

The axial CT images demonstrate centrilobular and peripheral nodules within the lung, worse in the mid zones. In addition there is mediastinal and hilar lymphadenopathy. There is central lung scarring and retraction. These lung parenchymal appearances are typical for advanced sarcoidosis.

Sarcoid is a multisystem disorder characterised by noncaseating granulomas. It is most common in African-Caribbean females in the age group 20–40 years. Cardiac sarcoidosis is one of the least common manifestations of sarcoid. Only 5–10% of patients are symptomatic.

Sarcoidosis can be an incidental finding on an ECG or else clinical presentation can be due to arrhythmias, heart block, congestive heart failure, angina, ventricular aneurysm and, rarely, constrictive pericarditis or sudden death. The features of the disease are:
- Commonly involves the LV.
- Focal myocardial thickening.
- Delayed mid wall or transmural enhancement.

Sarcoid more commonly involves myocardium than pericardium, with relative sparing of the endocardium. There is a predisposition for the left ventricular lateral wall, basal septum and right ventricular free wall.

Cardiac sarcoidosis has three histopathological stages, all of which can potentially be visualised with cardiac MRI. Initial oedema is followed by granulomatous infiltration, with eventual progression to postinflammatory scarring. Spin-echo T2-weighted images will demonstrate oedema as areas of high signal intensity within the myocardium. Active granulomas may manifest as focal nodular areas on cine images. The myocardial fibrosis shows delayed enhancement on inversion recovery gradient-echo T1-weighted images – this is a sign of advanced disease and is a poor prognostic factor. Scarring will appear as focal areas of thinning with associated hypokinesia and delayed enhancement in a nonvascular territory affecting the subepicardial layer, typically affecting the basal and lateral left ventricular segments. Patients with advanced cardiac sarcoid are prone to cardiac arrhythmias and sudden death and right ventricular late gadolinium enhancement can predict the need for ICD placement.

**ii.** Pulmonary findings include bilateral hilar lymphadenopathy, reticulonodular opacities, nodules along the fissures/bronchovascular bundles and fibrosis (15d, e).

## QUESTION 16

**16** A 27-year-old female was referred to the cardiology clinic by her obstetrician because of symptoms of breathlessness on minimal exertion. The patient was in her 18th week of gestation and this was her first pregnancy. She grew up in India until the age of 16 years and had had rheumatic fever as a child. Her routine blood results showed that she was not anaemic. On examination, she was in sinus rhythm with a mid diastolic murmur. Her transthoracic echocardiogram showed that she has severe mitral stenosis with a mitral orifice area calculated at 0.8 cm². No evidence of intracardiac shunts was detected. A CXR showed that her lung fields were clear. Following a detailed discussion about risks and benefits, a decision was made to proceed with PTMC (16). A TOE was scheduled prior to her PTMC.

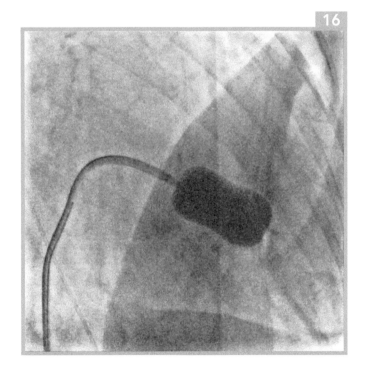

i. What is PTMC?

ii. Why is a TOE necessary prior to PTMC?

iii. What is the long-term success rate of PTMC?

## Answer 16

**16i.** PTMC, also known as percutaneous mitral balloon valvotomy, was first performed in the 1980s. There have been some refinements in the techniques over the years and today the most common technique uses an hourglass-shaped single balloon called the Inoue balloon. PTMC is a Class I recommendation for symptomatic patients with moderate–severe mitral stenosis with favourable valve morphology (pliable, noncalcified valve without significant subvalvular disease). It is also a Class I recommendation for asymptomatic patients with moderate–severe mitral stenosis and favourable valve morphology who have severe pulmonary hypertension (pulmonary artery systolic pressure >50 mmHg at rest or >60 mmHg with exercise). A PTMC procedure is performed via the right femoral vein and requires a trans-septal puncture (atrial septostomy) to gain access to the left heart. Once the uninflated Inoue balloon is positioned across the stenosed mitral valve, it is inflated and assumes an hourglass shape. This unique shape allows the balloon to centre on the mitral valve at its 'waist' preventing it from migrating during the process of inflation. In this case, the fully inflated Inoue balloon is shown in the fluoroscopic image (16). The immediate results of PTMC are usually fairly impressive, with an average doubling of mean valve area and a 50% reduction in the transmitral gradient.

**ii.** The presence of left atrial thrombus and significant mitral regurgitation are contraindications to PTMC. If an intracardiac clot is identified, formal anticoagulation will be required for a number of weeks until complete clot dissolution, before PTMC can be considered. The presence of significant mitral regurgitation precludes PTMC because balloon inflation of the mitral valve is likely to worsen the degree of regurgitation. In these patients with significant mitral regurgitation, the approach should be surgical mitral valve replacement. A TOE requested in this patient prior to PTMC was therefore to exclude the presence of left atrial thrombus and to exclude the presence of moderate–severe mitral regurgitation.

**iii.** It has been shown that 80% of patients who have had PTMC do not require reintervention 5 years after the procedure. One of the main determinants of success is the experience of the operator, so this procedure should only be performed at high volume centres.

17  A 48-year-old female was admitted to hospital with dyspnoea, chest pain and a feeling of pressure on her chest. A CXR was ordered as part of her investigations (17). The patient had had a normal CXR 5 months previously with a normal heart size.

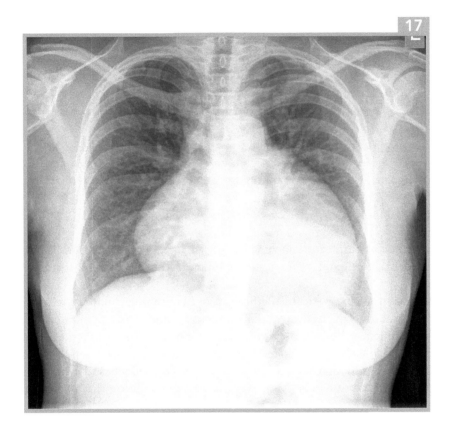

i.    What is the diagnosis?

ii.   Does cardiac tamponade only occur with a large volume of pericardial fluid?

## Answer 17

**17i.** The CXR shows globular enlargement of the cardiac shadow. The lungs and pleural spaces are clear. The differentials include pericardial effusion, cardiac chamber enlargement or cardiomyopathy. In this case, as the patient had a normal CXR 5 months prior, the most likely diagnosis is a pericardial effusion. A globular appearance to the cardiac outline has been described with pericardial effusions, but the most useful sign is a rapid change in heart size or shape with little or no evidence of pulmonary venous congestion. Diagnosis is usually confirmed by echocardiography.

The heart is contained within the pericardium, which has visceral and parietal layers. Between these layers is the pericardial space which normally contains 15–30 ml of fluid. A pericardial effusion is an abnormal amount of fluid in the pericardial space.

Causes of pericardial effusion include:
- Infective: bacterial, viral (coxsackie virus A and B, HIV), fungal and TB.
- Malignant: metastatic commonly from lung, breast and leukaemia/lymphoma.
- Iatrogenic: postsurgical.
- Idiopathic.

Other less common causes include post-traumatic, nephrotic syndrome, myxoedema, aortic dissection, systemic lupus erythematosus and drugs.

Fluid analysis of the pericardial effusion can help in determining the cause. Fluid may be evaluated for lactic acid dehydrogenase, total protein, white cell count, Gram stain and cultures, TB culture, haematocrit and tumour markers. Symptoms from a pericardial effusion include dyspnoea, chest pain, pressure symptoms, hoarse voice (due to phrenic nerve compression), light-headedness and syncope. Treatment of pericardial effusion is based on the underlying condition that is causing it.

**ii.** No. Clinical manifestations are dependent upon the *rate* of accumulation of fluid in the pericardial sac. Cardiac tamponade may occur even with a small volume of pericardial fluid, if it has accumulated rapidly.

Cardiac tamponade can be a life threatening condition due to diastolic heart failure, reduced stroke volume and shock. It may occur following chest trauma, myocardial rupture (after MI) and heart surgery. On examination, the classic Beck triad of hypotension, muffled heart sounds and jugular venous distension should be sought. Another sign is pulsus paradoxus (a decrease in systolic blood pressure of more than 10 mmHg with inspiration). The diagnostic modality of choice is echocardiography. Treatment is by pericardiocentesis by which fluid is aspirated, commonly under ultrasound guidance. Alternatively, pericardial effusions can be drained surgically by a pericardial window.

# QUESTION 18

18   A 74-year-old male with a known past medical history of two previous myocardial
     infarctions with CABG and stent insertion, presents with further episodes of chest pain.
     A nuclear medicine MIBI scan was requested to look for evidence of reversible ischaemia.

i.    What does the test show (18)?

ii.   What is the average radiation dose from this examination?

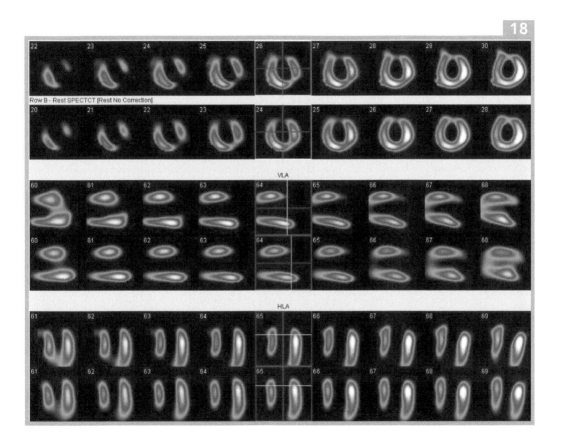

## Answer 18

**18i.** The MIBI scan shows a defect in the apical and anterior walls of the LV. This is identified on both the stress and rest images, which indicates that this is a fixed defect consistent with a previous infarct. There is no evidence here of reversible ischaemia. Appearances are therefore consistent with a LAD territory infarct. The patient was managed medically, with an increase in his antianginal medication.

**ii.** The combined dose of a MIBI scan (stress and rest component) is approximately 12 mSv which is a dose approximately equivalent to a CT abdomen investigation or approximately 600 CXRs. Background environmental radiation is approximately 3.0 mSv per year, so the examination would equate to 4 years of background radiation.

(Wall BF, Hart D. Revised radiation doses for typical x-ray examinations. *British Journal of Radiology* 1997;**70**:437–439.

## QUESTION 19

19  A 50-year-old female presents with sudden onset of dyspnoea and orthopnoea. On examination, there was dullness to percussion at the left base and basal crackles. She had a history of hypertension and ischaemic heart disease. A CXR was obtained. The patient also complained of chest pain and a raised D–dimer was found. She also had a history of malignancy and a pulmonary embolus was suspected. Selected images from the CT pulmonary angiogram are shown (which did not show a pulmonary embolus).

i.   What are the CXR (19a) and CT (19b, c) findings?

ii.  List some of the cardiac causes.

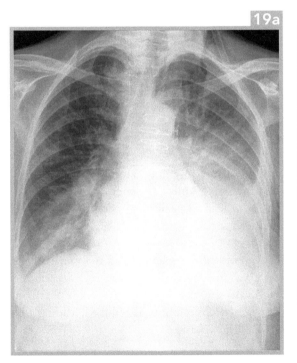

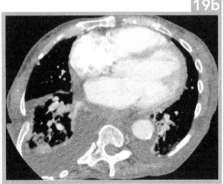

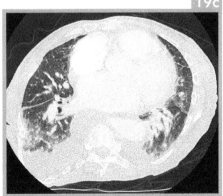

**19i.** The CXR shows a moderate sized left-sided pleural effusion, upper lobe venous diversion and perihilar consolidation. The heart size is difficult to comment upon since the radiograph is an AP film. Appearances are consistent with alveolar pulmonary oedema. The CT shows small bilateral pleural effusions, patchy ground-glass opacity and smooth interlobular septal thickening. The LV also appears dilated.

**ii.** Heart failure is a physiological state that occurs when the heart fails to pump an adequate cardiac output to meet the needs of the body. Cardiac causes of heart failure include ischaemic heart disease, hypertension, valvular disease and cardiomyopathies. Rarer causes include viral myocarditis, HIV cardiomyopathy, amyloid and alcohol.

There are several different ways to classify heart failure including left heart failure *vs.* right heart failure, systolic *vs.* diastolic dysfunction and the degree of functional impairment.

In left-sided heart failure, the LV fails to pump blood adequately into the systemic circulation and pulmonary venous pressure rises. Pulmonary oedema ensues with leakage of fluid into the pulmonary interstitium, alveoli and pleural space. Left-sided heart failure often presents with respiratory symptoms such as dyspnoea, orthopnoea and paroxysmal nocturnal dyspnoea.

Right-sided heart failure is most commonly caused by longstanding LV failure. The RV fails to pump blood adequately into the pulmonary circulation leading to increased systemic venous pressure. This may lead to peripheral oedema, ascites and hepatomegaly. However, mixed presentations are common.

In diastolic dysfunction, the ventricle has reduced compliance and is abnormally stiff. The result is a reduced end-diastolic volume, even though the end-diastolic pressure may be high. This leads to a reduced stroke volume by the Frank Starling mechanism. In systolic dysfunction, ventricular contractility is reduced, leading to a lower stroke volume at any given end-diastolic volume.

Heart failure can be classified according to the NYHA functional classification system, listed below:
- Class I: no limitation is experienced in any activities; there are no symptoms from ordinary activities.
- Class II: slight, mild limitation of activity; the patient is comfortable at rest or with mild exertion.
- Class III: marked limitation of any activity; the patient is comfortable only at rest.
- Class IV: any physical activity brings on discomfort and symptoms occur at rest.

## QUESTION 20

20 A 39-year-old female with a persistent fever over the last week was admitted to the accident and emergency department feeling lethargic and unwell. On examination, she was pyrexial, tachypnoeic and tachycardic. Cardiac auscultation revealed a grade 3/6 pansystolic murmur heard loudest at the apex radiating to the axilla. This has not been previously documented. Her inflammatory markers were elevated with a C-reactive protein of 228 mg/l and a white cell count of $18 \times 10^9$/l. Urine dipstick demonstrated evidence of microscopic haematuria. Blood cultures were obtained. She was referred for a TTE in view of the new murmur.

i. What does the echocardiographic image (20a) show?

ii. What are the common complications of this condition?

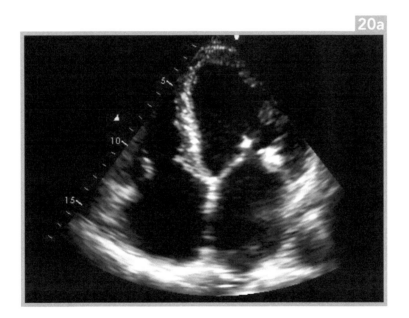

**20i.** In Figure 20b a large mass (arrow) can be seen attached to the posterior mitral valve leaflet, and given the clinical context, the most likely diagnosis is mitral valve endocarditis. Vegetation, abscess and new dehiscence of a prosthetic valve are the three major echocardiographic criteria for the diagnosis of infective endocarditis. A vegetation is an oscillating intracardiac mass attached to a valve, an endocardial structure or on implanted cardiac devices such as a pacing lead. The identification of vegetation can be made difficult when there are pre-existing valve abnormalities such as a thickened calcified valve or in the presence of mitral valve prolapse. Occasionally a papillary fibroelastoma can be confused as a vegetation, hence the clinical context is crucial. An abscess on echocardiography appears as a thickened, nonhomogenous perivalvular area which may appear either echodense or echolucent. Dehiscence of a prosthetic valve will appear as a paravalvular regurgitation which can be accompanied by rocking motion of the prosthesis. The sensitivity of TTE for diagnosing infective endocarditis is between 40% and 60%, and that of transoesophageal echocardiography is in excess of 90%. In cases when the initial study is negative, a repeat scan may be warranted in 1 week if the clinical suspicion remains high.

**ii.** The commonest complication of infective endocarditis is permanent damage to the valve structure, resulting in severe valvular regurgitation requiring surgical valve replacement. Valve damage can manifest amongst others as leaflet perforation, chordae rupture causing flail leaflet or valve aneurysm. Fistula formation can also develop between the different cardiac chambers and with the great vessels, for example between the aorta and the LA. If an aortic root abscess forms which extends into the septum, the conduction system may be disrupted and this may manifest as any degree of atrioventricular block on a 12-lead ECG.

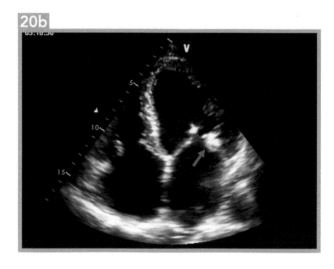

21   A 69-year-old male presents to his GP with an episode of slurring of speech which lasted for 12 hours and then resolved. The patient is a heavy smoker having smoked 60 cigarettes per day for 40 years. He had a single episode of haemoptysis 4 weeks previously and the GP was concerned about an underlying lung cancer with brain metastases and therefore referred him for an urgent CT chest. An ECG was performed in clinic and showed new AF. All blood tests including cardiac biomarkers were normal. Findings from the chest CT are shown (21).

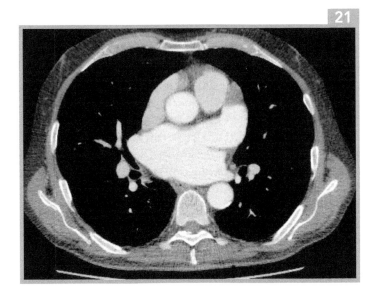

i.   What are the image findings?

ii.  What is the further management of this patient?

## Answer 21

**21i.** The axial image from a contrast enhanced CT scan, in arterial phase, demonstrates a filling defect in the left atrial appendage layered along the anterior wall. Given the clinical history and the CT appearance, the most likely diagnosis here is of thrombus in the LA as a consequence of AF. The patient's clinical history is that of a TIA secondary to a small embolus.

AF is the commonest arrhythmia and occurs when there is irregular conduction of impulses to the ventricles from another site, e.g. the pulmonary veins rather than from the sinoatrial node. AF is classified as:
- First detected – single episode.
- Paroxysmal – recurrent episodes which self terminate in fewer than 7 days.
- Persistent – recurrent episodes lasting more than 7 days.
- Permanent – long-term episode.

Clinical presentation can be variable but usually presents with palpitations. Other symptoms such as angina, dyspnoea, heart failure and syncope can also occur. Underlying causes include ischaemia, hyperthyroidism, mitral valve disease or it can be idiopathic. Investigation is via a 12-lead ECG or, if events are paroxysmal, then with a 24-hour ECG. Further investigation is with a transthoracic echocardiogram to exclude structural or functional heart disease and to assess cardiac function.

**ii.** Management requires either rhythm or rate control. Rhythm control is advised in lone and paroxysmal AF or in persistent AF in patients who are symptomatic; younger age group; secondary to a treated precipitant; or in patients with heart failure. Options for rhythm control are with electrical or pharmacological (e.g. sotalol, flecainide) cardioversion. In persistent AF, rate control should be performed in patients over 65 years; patients with coronary artery disease and in those who have contraindications to cardioversion or antiarrythmic drugs, e.g. digoxin.

Referral for specialist intervention, such as pulmonary vein isolation, pacemaker therapy, arrhythmia surgery, atrioventricular junction catheter ablation or use of atrial defibrillators, should be considered when pharmacological therapy has failed; in lone AF; and where there is evidence of an underlying electrophysiological disorder, e.g. Wolff–Parkinson–White syndrome.

Stroke assessment also needs to be carried out to determine whether the patient requires long-term anticoagulation with warfarin.

# QUESTION 22

22  A 31-year-old male presents to the emergency department having had a stroke. He has no past medical history and had previously been completely fit and well. He has never smoked and does not drink alcohol. All blood tests were normal.

i.   What is the diagnosis (22)?

ii.  Why is it important in young patients with stroke?

iii. What are the treatment options?

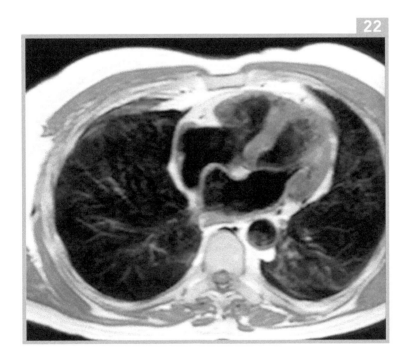

**22i.** A single axial MRI image has been provided which shows an ASA. ASA is a congenital abnormality of the atrial septum causing a localised saccular abnormality usually at the level of the fossa ovalis. There is oscillation or aneurysmal protrusion/bulging of the interatrial septum into either or both atria. The size of the base of the aneurysm should be more than 15 mm and should not involve the entire septum. The incidence is <1% on TTE.

**ii.** This diagnosis is of clinical importance because of its association with patent fossa ovalis, ASD and cryptogenic stroke. Approximately 70% patients have associated PFO and a 33% increase in the incidence of stroke. The incidence of stroke in patients with ASA and PFO is 3.8% compared with 1% without these anomalies. In young patients with stroke, ASA should be suspected as a cardioembolic source.

Patients with both ASA and PFO who have had a stroke are at increased risk of further strokes despite being on antiplatelet therapy. The proposed likely mechanism of the stroke is via formation of thrombus in the ASA with a paradoxical embolism through a PFO. Coughing and Valsalva manoeuvre can result in transient elevation of RA pressures and allows paradoxical emboli to pass from RA to LA through the PFO. In patients with both ASA and PFO the paradoxical emboli are due to preferential orientation of blood flow from the inferior vena cava towards the foramen ovale, due to the abnormal motion of the fossa ovalis membrane.

In some patients there is possible perforation of the ASA resulting in ASD and increased risk of paradoxical embolism.

ASAs are associated with supraventricular tachyarrhythmias like atrial fibrillation, mitral valve prolapse, PFO and migraines with aura. The diagnosis is usually established with transoesophageal echocardiography.

The Hanley criteria for diagnosis require aneurysmal dilatation of atrial septum protruding at least 15 mm beyond the plane of the atrial septum. The Olivares–Reyes criteria is a classification system based on the extent of excursion into each atrium.

Dynamic MRI studies are very useful in making the diagnosis of an ASA. The diagnostic feature of ASA on MRI is oscillation of the atrial septum into one or both atria throughout the cardiac cycle. The septum bulges into the LA at end systole, moves to midline at mid diastole and bulges into the RA at end diastole. A measurement of the base of the aneurysm and excursion into the atrium can be measured accurately on MRI.

**iii.** Isolated ASAs without any complications need regular follow up to look for thrombus in the aneurysm. No specific treatment is needed. Patients with ASA and associated PFO/ASD are treated medically with antiplatelet therapy, anticoagulants and surgical or percutaneous closure of the defect. In the presence of a shunt, to prevent recurrent paradoxical embolism, closure of the shunt is suggested.

## QUESTION 23

23  A patient who had a permanent pacemaker implanted 6 weeks previously for complete heart block attended the accident and emergency department with a syncopal episode. She had her pacemaker interrogated and it was noted that her ventricular lead was malfunctioning, suggesting that the lead might have displaced. A CXR was requested to look at the lead positions.

**i.** What does the CXR show (23a)?

**ii.** What are the causes of pacemaker lead displacement?

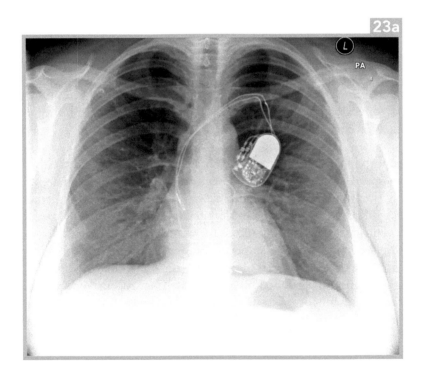

**23i.** The CXR shows that the ventricular lead has migrated, with the ventricular lead (23b, arrow) forming a loop within the right ventricular outflow tract/pulmonary artery.

**ii.** Pacemaker lead displacements occur most commonly in the early postimplantation period. Historic data from the early 1990s place the incidence of early lead displacement at about 5% for dual-chamber pacemakers and 1% for VVI pacemakers, with atrial leads being more commonly displaced (3.8% of cases) compared to ventricular leads (1.4%). With the advent of active fixation leads and improved awareness and experience, the incidence has declined but remains a problem. Lead displacement may be caused by poor lead placement with insufficient 'slack'. In such a scenario, the lead tends to move with deep inspiration, coughing or a change in body posture, increasing the risk of displacement and hence pacemaker malfunction. In some patients, lead displacement may be due to 'twiddler's syndrome', a condition describing patients who, whether consciously or subconsciously, fiddle with the pulse generator, twisting it around. Over time, with constant twisting of the pulse generator, the leads may be pulled up by traction and not commonly the leads have been found outwith the heart, i.e. within the superior vena cava (23c, arrows, different patient).

In a proportion of cases where the leads are optimally placed, excessive physical activity, especially involving the ipsilateral arm to the pulse generator, during the early postimplantation phase can cause unexpected lead displacement. Most cardiology departments aim for an 'acceptable' lead displacement rate of less than 1% for ventricular leads and no more than 2–3% for atrial leads. Not uncommonly, microdisplacements of leads can occur (as opposed to macrodisplacements), i.e. when no radiological evidence of displacement is seen but the lead has obviously displaced as it no longer functions appropriately on pacemaker interrogation. Whether it is micro- or macrodisplacement, lead repositioning is required and often an active fixation lead is used to achieve a more stable position.

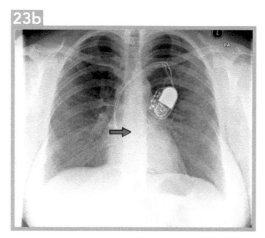

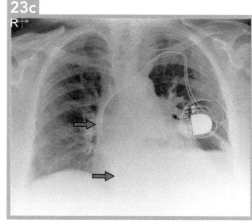

## QUESTION 24

24 A 40-year-old female presents with acute SOB, widespread T-wave inversion, positive troponin test and her CXR shows normal cardiac silhouette but perihilar interstitial shadowing. TTE showed globally poor ventricular function but initial catheter coronary angiogram showed no significant stenosis and the patient recovered after a short coronary care unit admission. TTE 6 months later showed markedly improved ventricular function.

i.   What are the differentials for this history? What is the key feature on these images that distinguishes these findings (24a, b)?

ii.  What is the most common cause for this condition and what is the usual prognosis?

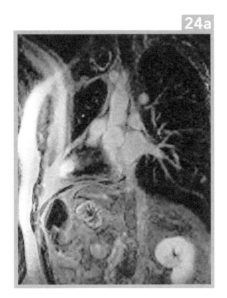

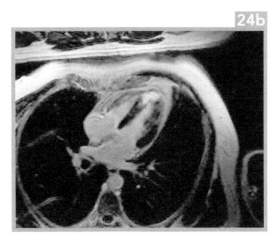

## Answer 24

**24i.** The history describes acute cardiac decompensation, with 'flash pulmonary oedema', confirmed by poor function on TTE, which would be compatible with acute MI given the troponin rise. However, the coronary arteries are normal on gold-standard catheter angiogram. The most likely differential for this situation is infective myocarditis.

Cardiac MRI can be very useful in differentiating between ischaemia and myocarditis. Although both ischaemia and myocarditis can result in focal wall motion abnormality, they differ in appearance on late gadolinium imaging. In ischaemia there is subendocardial enhancement which can extend to become transmural. In myocarditis however, the late gadolinium enhancement is globular and intramyocardial and spares the subendocardium. Late gadolinium enhancement can last for 6–24 months in myocarditis.

**ii.** Myocarditis can be generally classified as infectious, autoimmune, drug-induced or post-transplant. Various chemotherapy agents and amphetamine analogues have been associated with myocarditis, which is often only partially reversible on cessation. There are many similarities in the imaging and pathology findings of autoimmune and chronic infectious myocarditis, presumably relating to the immune response to internalised viral markers within infected myocytes. Although many infectious agents are known to cause myocarditis, the most common is viral and in those cases in which no cause is found, a viral agent is generally presumed to be the cause.

Prognosis depends on the presentation, with a fulminant presentation associated with a markedly better outcome (near normal), if they survive the initial period of infection without transplant. The more indolent the infection, the more severe the LV impairment and worse the mortality. Factors which indicate a worse prognosis are syncope, severe LV impairment (<25%) and heart block.

Cocaine-related myopathy is a possible differential in a patient with the above clinical history and normal coronary arteries. It is caused in two ways, the first via multiple vasospasm-induced infarcts and the second via a poorly understood pathway, involving chronic adrenergic stimulation and associated with marked increase in LV myocardial mass. The key feature to exclude cocaine-related infarct is the lack of subendocardial late gadolinium enhancement. Note also the normal thickness of the LV myocardium.

# QUESTION 25

25 A 41-year-old male presents to the emergency department with acute onset of chest pain. He has no cardiovascular risk factors and at presentation has a normal ECG, a negative troponin, and normal CXR. He has a TIMI score of 0 and a GRACE score of <3. He was managed conservatively and an out-patient cardiac CT was organised.

i.   What does the cardiac CT show (25a–c)?

ii.  What would be the appropriate further management for this patient?

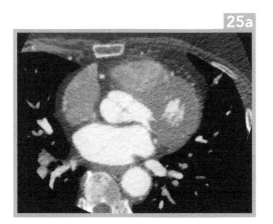

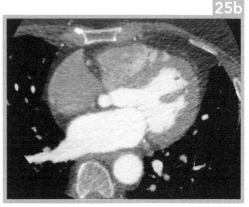

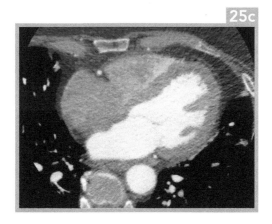

## Answer 25

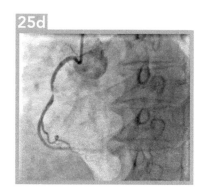

**25i.** Selected axial images from the cardiac CT investigation show evidence of a short significant stenosis in the mid RCA and appearances would be consistent with a significant lesion here. Stenoses on CT are commonly reported in a similar way to that on invasive angiography such that minimal stenosis is <25% luminal narrowing; mild is 25–50%; moderate is 50–70% and significant is >70%. In this case there is a >50% diameter reduction which corresponds to a >75% stenosis.

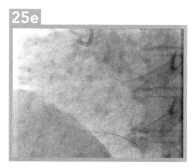

On CT it is possible to make an attempt at classifying the type of atherosclerotic plaques. Plaques can be divided into calcified and noncalcified/soft plaques. The CT attenuation of noncalcified plaques may help towards plaque characterisation – attenuation within fibrous plaques (75–120 HU) is usually higher than within lipid-rich fatty plaques (10–90 HU). It is thought that highly lipid-rich plaques with very low CT attenuation values of <30 HU have an increased risk of plaque rupture.

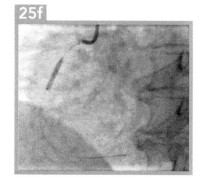

**ii.** This is a solitary significant lesion within the RCA and therefore further management involves urgent referral for an invasive angiogram +/- angioplasty. There is excellent correlation between cardiac CT findings and invasive angiography, with cardiac CT diagnosing coronary artery disease with 99% sensitivity, 96% specificity, 87% positive predictive value and 100% negative predictive value.

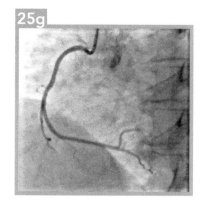

Figures 25d–g demonstrate the further management of the patient, with the lesion confirmed on invasive angiogram and treatment with angioplasty and stent insertion.

26  A 56-year-old male who had a mechanical St. Jude bileaflet aortic valve prosthesis replaced 3 years ago presents to hospital with symptoms of exertional breathlessness and atypical chest pain. His troponin level was mildly elevated but there were no dynamic ECG changes. He was referred for in-patient coronary angiography in view of his presumed acute coronary syndrome. No flow-limiting coronary artery stenosis was found.

i.   What does the fluoroscopy image show (26a)?

ii.  What is a bileaflet mechanical aortic valve?

iii. What is important to elicit from the history given the fluoroscopic findings?

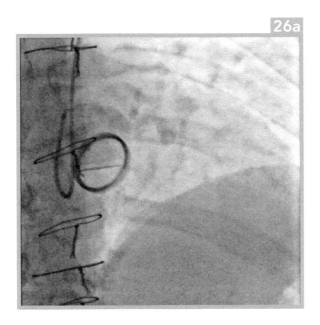

## Answer 26

**26i.** The fluoroscopic image was obtained from a near en-face projection with the radiographic beam being almost perpendicular to the valve plane. During systole when the leaflets of a mechanical bileaflet valve are fully tilted in the open position, fluoroscopy should reveal two radio-opaque 'lines' across the ring, with both lines positioned just lateral to the central axis. Each line represents a leaflet. This fluoroscopic image only shows one line (26b, arrow) suggesting that one of the leaflets is stuck in the 'closed' position, hence causing valve obstruction. This would explain the patient's presenting symptoms of exertional breathlessness.

**ii.** A bileaflet mechanical aortic valve prosthesis consists of two semicircular rigid leaflets attached to a ring (26c). The leaflets pivot at two hinges located slightly lateral to the central axis of the valve. When the leaflets are in the 'open' position as shown, the leaflets are almost perpendicular to the valve plane and an en-face fluoroscopic image should demonstrate two radio-opaque lines. Transvalvular forward flow is via two large lateral semicircular orifices and a narrow rectangular central orifice. The leaflets can often open up to 80 degrees.

**iii.** Compliance to anticoagulant treatment needs to be ascertained. The most common cause of prosthetic valve obstruction is subtherapeutic anticoagulation leading to valve thrombosis. Often the clinical history would reveal that the patient had stopped their anticoagulation for an invasive procedure, e.g. endoscopy or minor surgical procedures, while receiving inadequate cover with other antithrombotic agents such as unfractionated heparin. The first-line treatment for patients with confirmed valve thrombosis is thrombolytic therapy in the absence of any contraindications. The other possible cause of valve obstruction is pannus formation. Pannus is an abnormal overgrowth of tissue (almost like excessive scarring) which encroaches centripetally and, if significant, the valve leaflets can be immobilised resulting in valve obstruction. The definitive treatment in such patients is re-do surgery.

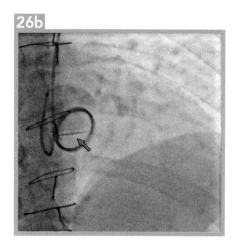

26b

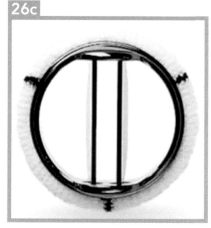

26c

27 A 65-year-old patient, a known diabetic, presents with increasing shortness of breath, now experienced on even mild exertion. This all started after an episode of mild chest pain 6 months ago, ascribed to indigestion by their GP. There is a past medical history of a TIA.

i.    What morphological features are present in the first two images (27a, b) to explain the patient's symptoms? What further feature is present in the right hemi-thorax?

ii.   Which cardiac segments are likely to be involved (27c) and what vessels are likely to be involved?

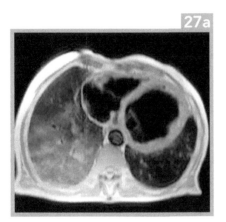

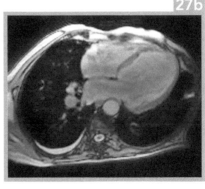

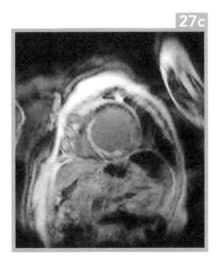

## Answer 27

**27i.** Figures 27a and 27b show a dilated LV, diffuse opacity in both lungs worse on the right and there is also a small right pleural effusion.

Myocardial infarction causes 12 million deaths each year worldwide and is the leading cause of death in industrialised countries. Classical presentation is of central chest pain, radiating to the left arm or neck and often associated with dizziness and shortness of breath. However, presentation is often nonclassical and may be occult in those patients with high pain thresholds, altered mental status/dementia or a disorder of angina nociception, such as diabetes mellitus. Features associated with a poorer prognosis include increasing age, diabetes, other vascular disease, delayed presentation and evidence LVF.

LVF causes impaired ability to meet systemic vascular supply and left-sided overload and increased pulmonary vein pressure, which, in turn leads to pulmonary oedema. Functional severity can be graded using the NYHA classification (see Question 19). Prognosis is poor for stage 4 disease, with an annual mortality between 10% and 20%.

Imaging features of LVF are a dilated LV and pulmonary oedema on CXR. On echocardiogram, there is dilatation of the LV, with hypo/akinesia and reduced ejection fraction (<55%). Similar features are seen on cardiac MRI as with echo, but additionally, stress and resting perfusion and late gadolinium enhancement can be demonstrated.

Myocardial stunning is a temporary impaired wall motion, which recovers without intervention. Myocardial hibernation is prolonged impaired wall motion but is reversible with appropriate revascularisation. Both stunning and hibernation cause a resting perfusion defect and are associated with regional wall hypo/akinesia but are not associated with LV wall thinning.

The major differential of focal hypo/akinesia or resting hypoperfusion is an established infarction of the myocardium, which has the potential to become arrhythmogenic on revascularisation. A key feature of infarction over hibernation is the presence of late gadolinium enhancement. This can be graded depending on the thickness of myocardium involved and the number of segments affected.

**ii.** In Figure 27c, clear late gadolinium enhancement is demonstrated in the mid inferior and inferoseptal segments, which is associated with myocardial thinning in the mid-to-apical segments on the long-axis views (27a, b). This is likely to correspond to LAD and RCA stenosis causing infarction to the affected segments.

# QUESTION 28

28  A 40-year-old female presents to accident and emergency with chest pain. A CXR was performed as part of the investigations (28).

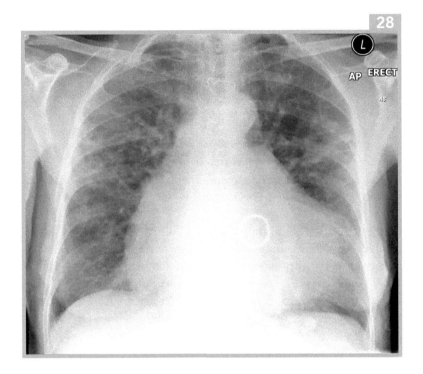

i.   Which cardiac valve has been replaced in this patient?

ii.  Which type of valve requires lifelong warfarin?

## Answer 28

**28i.** The chest radiographs show a mitral valve replacement. The heart appears enlarged despite AP projection and there is a double heart border indicative of LA enlargement. Other PA chest radiograph findings of LA enlargement include splaying of the carina and a prominent LA appendage.

**ii.** If the mitral valve is too damaged to permit repair then the valve must be replaced. Mitral valve replacement can be performed for mitral stenosis or mitral regurgitation.

There are two primary types of artificial mitral valves – a metal or mechanical valve and a tissue or biological valve. Mechanical valves require patients to take warfarin lifelong but have the advantage of better durability. Tissue valves do not require a patient to take warfarin, but only last 10–15 years. The patient's age, medical condition, preferences with medication and lifestyle are taken into consideration when deciding upon which type of valve is used.

Mitral stenosis is most commonly due to rheumatic fever. Other causes are congenital stenosis, amyloid, carcinoid, extensive mitral annular calcification and atrial myxoma. As the process worsens, mitral stenosis leads to raised LA pressure, pulmonary venous hypertension and eventually right ventricular failure. Cine MRI can be used to visualise the signal void jet arising from the mitral valve in diastole and enlargement of the LA and pulmonary venous hypertension. Velocity mapping can be used to estimate the transvalvular pressure gradient and for direct planimetry of the valve.

Mitral regurgitation is commonly due to myxomatous degeneration. Mitral regurgitation is also commonly due to ischaemic heart disease. (Myocardial infarction can lead to LV dilatation and enlargement of the valvular orifice. Infarction or rupture of a papillary muscle can also occur.) Other causes include rheumatic fever and endocarditis. Chronic mitral regurgitation leads to LA and LV volume overload. The LV dilates in order to maintain stroke volume. Pulmonary venous hypertension is usually less severe than with mitral stenosis. Cine MRI can demonstrate the signal void from the regurgitant jet. Velocity mapping allows the regurgitant fraction to be quantified.

# QUESTION 29

29  An elderly patient was rushed to hospital because of acute breathlessness. He had a 60–pack–year history of smoking and was only on amlodipine for hypertension. On examination, he was tachypnoeic and appeared undernourished. His blood pressure was noted to be 100/45 mmHg and he was tachycardic (110 bpm). His oxygen saturation was measured at 90% on room air. Chest auscultation revealed some reduced breath sounds over the right base with dullness to percussion. A CXR and a CT thorax were requested.

i.   What does the CXR show (29a)?

ii.  What does the CT image show (29b)?

iii. What are the causes of pericardial effusion?

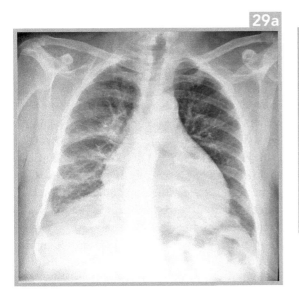

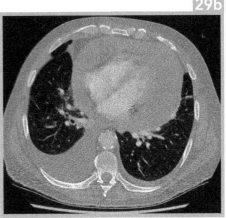

## Answer 29

**29i.** The CXR shows a globular cardiac silhouette and radiographic evidence of cardiomegaly. This was not noted previously. There was evidence of blunting of the right costophrenic angle and a suspicious spiculated lesion seen in the right mid zone.

**ii.** The CT image shows a large global pericardial effusion encompassing the heart. There is also a right-sided pleural effusion. In this patient, the spiculated mass on the CXR was later confirmed to be a primary lung cancer. The patient had an urgent pericardial drain inserted to remove the fluid which was compressing the heart and symptomatically the patient felt much better. The pericardial fluid was confirmed to be a malignant effusion.

**iii.** A large number of disease processes can affect the pericardium, including infections (viral, bacterial, fungal, parasitic), autoimmune diseases (collagen vascular diseases), malignant disease (primary or more commonly secondary causes), metabolic disorders (uraemia, myxoedema) and diseases that affect the myocardium predominantly, such as amyloidosis. All these conditions can cause a pericardial effusion. Additionally, a pericardial effusion can also be caused by bleeding into the pericardial space (haemopericardium) in situations such as a dissecting aortic aneurysm, trauma, in patients with clotting disorders or iatrogenic coronary perforation during percutaneous coronary intervention. Large effusions, such as in this case, are most common with malignancy-related effusion (35% due to a lung primary, 22% breast cancer and 18% leukaemia/lymphoma), tuberculous pericarditis and any cause of active bleeding into the pericardial space. The normal pericardial sac contains about 20–40 ml of pericardial fluid physiologically. If an effusion accumulates gradually over weeks and months, for example a malignant effusion, up to 1.5–2 litres of pericardial fluid may be present without haemodynamic compromise. However, if the effusion rapidly accumulates, as little as 250 ml is sufficient to cause circulatory collapse. In such a scenario, urgent pericardiocentesis is indicated. This is a percutaneous technique whereby a needle is inserted into the pericardial space under fluoroscopic and ultrasound guidance through a subxiphoid or apical approach. In patients who get recurrent effusions, a surgical pericardial window may be required, creating a link between the pericardial and pleural space. The prognosis of patients with pericardial effusion is dependent on aetiology and comorbid conditions.

# QUESTION 30

30 A 48-year-old female with hypertension, poor mobility and obesity presents to the accident and emergency department with atypical chest pain. She has a sinus tachycardia but no ST changes and has normal cardiac biomarkers. She also has a normal CXR. She continued to have pain and was getting progressively short of breath. There was significant clinical concern, and therefore a triple rule-out CT was requested (30a–d).

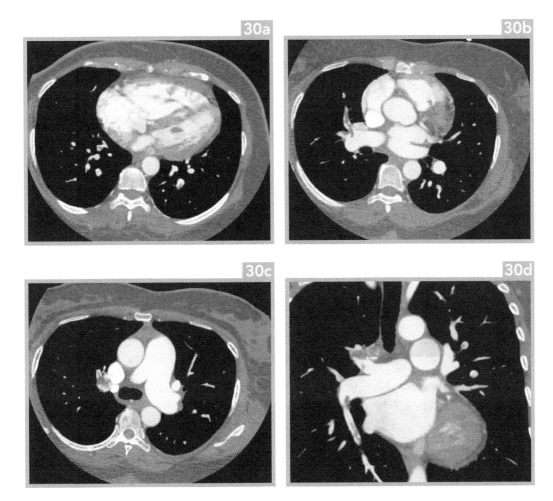

i.    What is the diagnosis?

ii.   How should the patient be managed?

## Answer 30

**30i.** Figures 30a–d are from a triple rule-out examination performed on an Aquilion One CT scanner which performs an up to 16 cm volume gated examination with a rotation of one-third of a second. The entire chest can therefore be covered in two volumes, with the images volumes then stitched together. In a triple rule-out examination the contrast well opacifies the pulmonary arteries, the aorta and the coronary arteries all in the same investigation, such that PEs, coronary artery disease and acute aortic pathologies, e.g. dissection, can be identified.

In this case the axial images demonstrate thrombus within the right main pulmonary artery with thrombus also seen within the right upper and lower lobe pulmonary arteries (better demonstrated on a coronal reformatted image – 30d). The axial images also demonstrate evidence of pulmonary artery hypertension and right ventricular strain, suggesting heavy embolus load and a poor prognosis.

PE is common and potentially lethal, affecting all ages. It accounts for >170,000 emergency admissions/year in England. It has a significant morbidity and mortality – by the age of 80 years, 11% of the population will have had a thromboembolic event. Three-month mortality rate is as high as 15%. PE is a significant cause of maternal death.

Ventilation/perfusion lung scintigraphy has a role in the investigation of PE if the CXR is normal. CTPA is now used as the 'gold standard' in the investigation of suspected PE.

**ii.** CTPA also allows assessment of the main pulmonary artery and the RV. Significant PEs have a poor morbidity and mortality – CT allows for assessment of the main pulmonary artery (considered dilated if it measures >2.9 cm, a sign of pulmonary artery hypertension) and also the RV (a ratio of RV/LV diameter of >1.5 is considered a poor prognostic sign). If there are features of haemodynamic instability or RV dysfunction, then consideration for thrombolysis should be made. If however the patient is stable with no RV strain, then monitoring, low molecular weight heparin and warfarin would be the management of choice.

# QUESTION 31

31 A 64-year-old male with a known history of well-controlled angina presents to his GP with gradually increasing symptoms, and on further questioning recalls that this deterioration started with a significant bout of angina chest pain ~6 months previously. He continues to smoke ~20 cigarettes per day; is overweight and has type 2 diabetes. He has also noted worsening shortness of breath and on examination has reduced breath sounds bibasally. The patient was referred for CT chest and also for a cardiology review. An invasive angiogram was performed.

i.  What does the invasive angiogram show (31a)?

ii. What does the CT show (31b)?

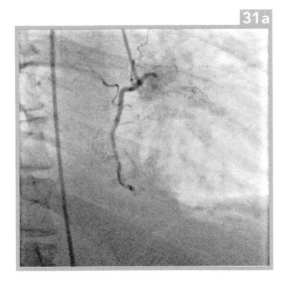

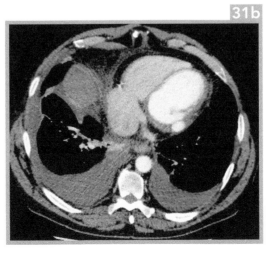

## Answer 31

**31i.** The invasive angiogram demonstrates a complete occlusion to the mid right coronary artery with a moderately diseased segment proximal to it. This looks like a chronically occluded lesion.

**ii.** The CT demonstrates two significant findings. Firstly, there are bilateral pleural effusions which in the presence of the angiographic findings would suggest a degree of heart failure. Secondly, there is a false aneurysm identified related to the posterolateral wall of the LV.

False aneurysm or pseudoaneurysms of the LV occurs when there is LV rupture which is contained by layers of pericardium/extracardiac tissue. In this case it will have occurred as a consequence of a myocardial infarction, which would fit with the clinical history given of an episode of severe chest pain 6 months previously. Trauma, postcardiac surgery and endocarditis are other causes of this type of aneurysm. Typically they are located in the posterolateral wall or the inferior wall of the LV. Differentiation from true aneurysms can be made by position; the size of the neck (false aneurysms have a very narrow neck); and the absence of covering myocardium. False aneurysms carry a significant risk of delayed rupture (which is not seen in true aneurysms) and therefore need surgical repair.

32 A 62-year-old female with CCS class III angina is seen in the cardiology clinic. She was referred for a coronary angiogram to assess the need for revascularisation as she was already on maximal medical therapy. There was a radiographically equivocal segment associated with some haziness seen in the distal LAD artery (32a, arrow). The severity of the stenosis was further assessed by IVUS (32b, c).

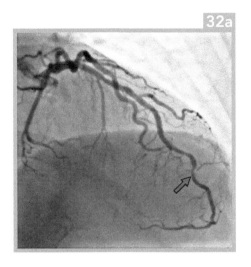

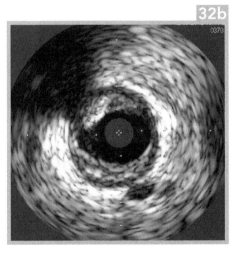

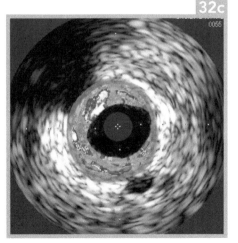

i. What does Figure 32b show?

ii. What is the principle underpinning IVUS?

## Answer 32

**32i.** Figure 32b shows a cross-section of the distal LAD where the equivocal segment was seen fluoroscopically. There is an obvious atheromatous plaque seen at the 2 o'clock position, resulting in an eccentric narrowing of the coronary lumen.

**ii.** IVUS is an emerging imaging modality that is employed in the setting of coronary angiography, i.e. in the cardiac catheterisation laboratory. An IVUS catheter consists of an ultrasound probe mounted on a flexible monorail tube that can be guided along an angioplasty wire into the coronary artery. Ultrasound frequencies of 10–45 MHz are emitted and the reflected signal is received and analysed, resulting in the generation of an image as shown (32b). Blood appears echolucent (i.e. black). The soft tissue features of the vessel wall are variably echo-opaque. Calcium reflects the most ultrasound, so areas with the brightest white represent calcification with an area of echo drop-out seen beyond it.

In clinical practice IVUS is useful in improving assessment of eccentric atheromatous plaque when standard angiographic images are equivocal. It is also utilised in patients who have left main stem disease to help in selecting the most appropriately sized stent diameter. It can also be used to check how well a stent has been deployed (stent apposition) following balloon inflation of an intracoronary stent. Stents that are underexpanded (i.e. not expanded flushed against the coronary artery wall) are at increased risk of stent thrombosis and stent restenosis. Further balloon dilatation of the stent is required until the stent is well apposed with the vessel wall. IVUS is also increasingly used to help the assessment of complex lesions, in particular complex bifurcation disease, to guide the interventionist in devising the best strategy for stenting. More recently, IVUS software has been developed to provide information about the composition of atheromatous plaques. This new functionality is also known as virtual histology. The relative composition of a plaque (lipid, calcium, fibrous tissue, necrotic material) can be qualitatively estimated with virtual histology, whereby the different tissue type and composition is represented by different colours. Green represents fibrous tissue, red necrotic tissue, yellow fibrofatty tissue and white calcium. Figure 32c shows the histological composition of the lesion in question using the virtual histology function. This is a predominantly fibrocalcific atheroma.

# QUESTION 33

33 A 36-year-old female presents with some pleuritic chest pain and shortness of breath after a recent lung infection and a 13-hour flight. Clinically she was felt to be at high risk of a PE and a CTPA was performed (33). There was no evidence of a PE and the symptoms were thought to be due to pleurisy. The scan however, was not entirely normal.

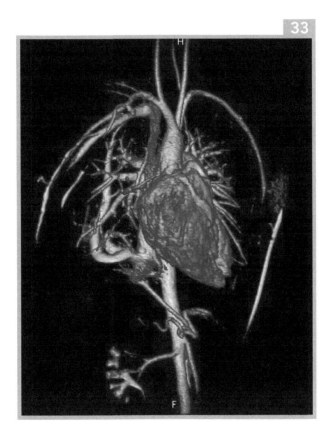

i.   What is the diagnosis?

ii.  How do patients present clinically?

iii. What are the salient radiological features?

## Answer 33

**33i.** Scimitar syndrome, also called hypogenetic lung syndrome or pulmonary venolobar syndrome, is a special form of partial anomalous pulmonary venous drainage where all of the right side pulmonary vessels drain a hypoplastic lung into a large vein which in turn drains into the IVC at the level of the diaphragm. This large vein resembles a Turkish scimitar sword, hence the name Scimitar syndrome. The number of anomalous veins involved determines the symptoms and signs. This is a left-to-right shunt.

There is a venous, an arterial and a pulmonary anomaly. The venous anomaly is abnormal drainage of the pulmonary veins into the right heart. The pulmonary abnormality can be a sequestered lobe of the lung or hypoplastic or aplastic right pulmonary artery, hypoplastic or absent bronchi. The lung is frequently perfused via the aorta.

This syndrome is more common in females, can be familial and usually involves the right lung. The left lung is very rarely involved. Other associations include ASD, VSD, PDA, TOF, pulmonary sequestration and malformations of the diaphragm. The clinical symptoms depend on the extent of left-to-right shunt. Approximately 40% of patients are asymptomatic, in whom it is discovered as an incidental finding on a PA chest radiograph.

**ii.** Clinical symptoms are usually age dependent. In newborns the presentation is with heart failure due to right heart volume overload and pulmonary hypertension. Older children usually present with pulmonary infections. Young adults present with fatigue and dyspnoea on exertion and recurrent lung infections. The symptoms also depend on the size of the shunt. Cyanosis develops due to Eissenmenger's syndrome.

**iii.** Diagnosis is usually made by transthoracic or transoesophageal echocardiography. CT and MRI give anatomical details.
- Echo shows anomalous pulmonary venous drainage into the right heart.
- CXR can show hypoplasia of the right lung, dextraposition of the heart due to the hypoplastic lung and sometimes even large curved scimitar vein.
- CT demonstrates the systemic arterial supply from the aorta. In Figure 33 the vascular 3D reconstructed image shows the right-sided pulmonary vessel draining into the IVC. It also shows a systemic arterial supply from the coeliac axis to a right lower lobe.

Surgical treatment should be considered in cases of significant left-to-right shunt and pulmonary hypertension. Treatment is by anastomosis of the pulmonary veins to the LA by creating an interatrial baffle, or reimplantation of the anomalous vein into the LA and embolisation of the atypical arterial supply.

Differential diagnosis includes pulmonary sequestration and unilateral absence of pulmonary artery.

# QUESTION 34

34   The images shown are from follow up MRI of a 16-year-old Caucasian male
     (34a–c). He is hypertensive and on examination has radiofemoral delay.

i.   What is the diagnosis?

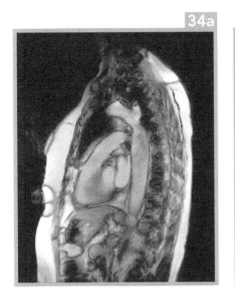

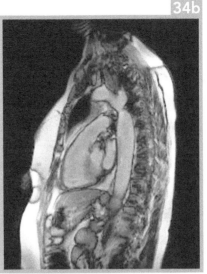

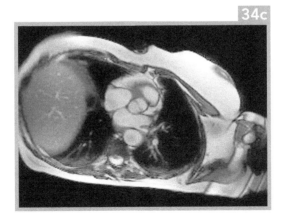

ii.  How can the functional significance be assessed?

## Answer 34

**34i.** Coarctation of the aorta.

Coarctation is a common congenital anomaly referring to narrowing of the aorta in the region of the ductus arteriosus. In adult coarctation, the area of narrowing tends to occur distal to the origin of the left subclavian artery (postductal). The condition usually does not cause symptoms in the neonatal period and is usually an incidental finding late in life. Preductal coarctation (occurring proximal to the ductus) is less common and usually presents in infancy. This type is associated with hypoplasia of the aortic arch.

With adult coarctation, coexistent cardiac anomalies are uncommon. With infantile coarctation, coexistent cardiac anomalies such as bicuspid valve (34c) (25–50%), PDA (33%), VSD (15%), aortic stenosis and aortic insufficiency, ASD, truncus arteriosis and double outlet RV occur. Turner's syndrome is associated in 13–15% of cases.

**ii.** Gradient-echo and velocity mapping techniques can be utilised to assess the functional significance of coarctation of the aorta. Gradient-echo may demonstrate abnormal flow as a signal void arising from the site of coarctation. With velocity mapping, blood flow velocity across the stenosis can be measured and the pressure gradient estimated using the modified Bernoulli equation. A resting peak velocity of greater than 3 m/s is significant.

Haemodynamically significant lesions are associated with the development of collaterals mainly from the intercostal arteries (leading to inferior rib notching on chest radiograph). Collateralisation may also occur from the internal mammary and anterior spinal arteries, for example. With increasing severity of stenosis and therefore increasing collateralisation, flow over the stenosis may decrease and velocities may normalise. Therefore, additional quantification of collateral flow is recommended in the evaluation of coarctation in order to provide a more direct assessment of the haemodynamic significance. This is done by measuring the inflow into the stenosis by a plane orientated orthogonal through the aorta, just proximal to the stenosis. Aortic flow at the level of the diaphragm is also measured. In normal individuals, the distal aortic flow is approximately 7% lower than that in the proximal aorta. An increase in flow >5% at the distal site is highly indicative of the presence of collateral flow.

# QUESTION 35

35 A 28-year-old Caucasian female was rushed to the emergency department with central chest pain with a typical distribution for ischaemic cardiac pain. She has always been physically fit and works as an investment banker with no significant past medical history. She was not on any regular medications. There was no family history of ischaemic heart disease. She has just returned from a long-haul flight from Australia the day before her admission to hospital. She vehemently denies any recreational drug use. A 12-lead ECG showed that she has significant ST elevation of her inferior leads but the ST elevation was however transient, i.e. dynamic. Following a brief discussion with the cardiology team, she had emergent coronary angiography. Figure 35 shows the fluoroscopic finding following contrast injection into the right coronary artery.

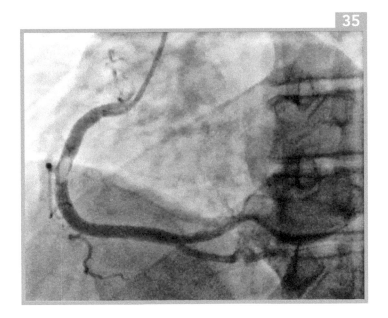

i. What is the likely cause for the patient's chest pain?

ii. What are the treatment strategies for this patient?

iii. What further tests will she require in the next few days?

**35i.** Coronary embolism is a rare clinical cause of acute myocardial infarction. It should be suspected in young patients who do not have the traditional risk factors for developing ischaemic heart disease. Pathophysiologically, coronary embolism is distinct from conventional acute myocardial infarction in that the latter is due to acute atherosclerotic plaque rupture while the former is due to migration of an embolus into the coronary arterial system. Common causes for coronary embolism are infective endocarditis, prosthetic heart valve, cardiomyopathy with mural thrombus, arrhythmia which predisposes to thrombus formation, such as atrial fibrillation, and paradoxical embolisation through a PFO. The diagnosis is further supported if normal coronary arteries are confirmed on coronary angiography, with the only abnormality being the presence of unexpected thrombus within a coronary artery. Following clot removal, treatment is aimed at the underlying cause.

ii. The thrombus can be aspirated using a thrombus aspiration catheter. Thrombus aspiration can be performed on its own or, if the thrombus burden is felt to be large, a distal embolic protection device can be used to allow collection of any small emboli that may get showered downstream during thrombus aspiration. In this patient, it was felt the embolus was too large relative to the catheter size for thrombus aspiration. There was a risk of the embolus dislodging within the aorta during thrombus retrieval. The patient was instead started on a glycoprotein IIb/IIIa inhibitor infusion overnight and brought back for repeat coronary angiography. On repeat angiography, the coronary embolus had completely dissolved. The underlying coronary artery was smooth with no evidence of plaque disease.

iii. Echocardiography to assess for PFO/ASD, intracardiac thrombus and valvular disease; thrombophilia screen to assess for prothrombotic conditions; Doppler ultrasound of her leg veins to assess for the presence of deep vein thrombosis.

# QUESTION 36

36 A 61-year-old female with no cardiac risk factors presents with atypical chest pain. She attempted an exercise tolerance test but was unable to manage more than 2 minutes due to arthritis in her knees. A cardiac CT was performed (36a).

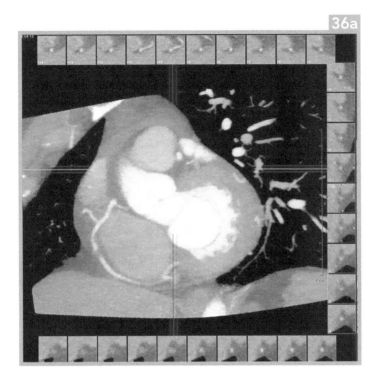

i. What does the cardiac CT show?

ii. Where does cardiac CT fit into the investigative pathway for new-onset chest pain according to the 2010 NICE guidelines?

**36i.** The cardiac CT demonstrates a significant soft plaque stenosis measuring ~1 cm in the mid RCA which is followed by a ~1 cm, long soft plaque subtotal occlusion of the mid RCA. The stenoses are particularly well demonstrated on the true axial reconstructions, which are arranged around the main image. These show no contrast in the RCA at the level of the subtotal occlusion (bottom row) and the significant stenosis (right row). The abnormalities were confirmed on invasive angiogram (36b) and the patient went on to have an angioplasty and stent insertion.

**ii.** In people without confirmed CAD, in whom stable angina cannot be diagnosed or excluded based on clinical assessment alone, estimate the likelihood of CAD. Take the clinical assessment and the resting 12-lead ECG into account when making the estimate. Arrange further diagnostic testing as follows:
- If the estimated likelihood of CAD is 61–90%, offer invasive coronary angiography as the first-line diagnostic investigation if appropriate.
- If the estimated likelihood of CAD is 30–60%, offer functional imaging as the first-line diagnostic investigation. When offering noninvasive functional imaging for myocardial ischaemia use:
  - MPI with SPECT *or*
  - stress echocardiography *or*
  - first-pass contrast-enhanced magnetic resonance perfusion *or*
  - MRI for stress-induced wall motion abnormalities.
- If the estimated likelihood of CAD is 10–29%, offer CT calcium scoring as the first-line diagnostic investigation. If the calcium score is:
  - zero, consider other causes of chest pain.
  - 1–400, offer 64-slice (or above) CT coronary angiography.
  - >400, offer invasive coronary angiography. If this is not clinically appropriate or acceptable to the person and revascularisation is not being considered, offer noninvasive functional imaging.
  - Do not use exercise ECG to diagnose or exclude stable angina for people without known CAD.

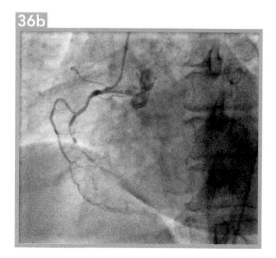

36b

This case however does demonstrate one of the flaws of the NICE guidelines since this patient had a calcium score of zero. The plaque was a noncalcified significant stenosis which would have been missed if the NICE guidelines had been followed.

# QUESTION 37

37 A 55-year-old patient presents with progressively worsening shortness of breath which appears to be worse with mobilising. Poor views were obtained on transthoracic echocardiography. CMR was requested to assess function.

i. What is the most important finding in the images (37a, b)?

ii. What additional features may be evident, and thus looked for, on CMR?

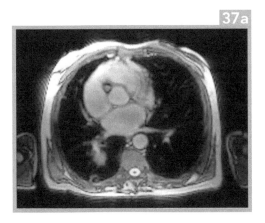

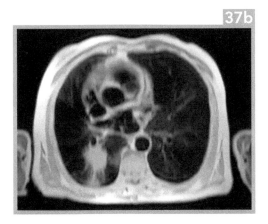

**37i.** The axial images demonstrate an incidental finding of a spiculated lesion in the right lower lobe which has the appearances of a primary bronchogenic carcinoma.

Incidental lung cancers are a rare finding on cardiac imaging, especially in centres which do not report full field of view images on cardiac CT. One recent study quoted figures of 0.3% incidental lung cancer findings on CT, of which 87% were not visible on the limited view images.

Discussion as to the merits of full field of view reporting relate to the high rate of incidental and benign pulmonary nodules, requiring further CT follow up and thus increased radiation dose. Current thinking states that nodules under 4 mm do not require formal follow up, unless there are features that increase the likelihood of malignancy, such as lymphadenopathy or adjacent pleural effusion.

**ii.** With CMR, the full field of view images should always be available and reported and these are usually the 'black-blood' gradient recalled-echo images. Although contrast enhancement can be seen on MRI, dedicated imaging of incidental pulmonary parenchymal lesions is not advised as CT provides a much clearer spatial resolution for determining extension and size (37c). The additional features of pleural effusions and lymphadenopathy can also be demonstrated.

The interval and number of follow up scans depends on the size of nodule and smoking risk, with more scans required for larger nodules in those with a significant smoking history. Benign features include well-defined, nonspiculated borders and coarse calcifications within the nodule.

Staging CT includes portovenous phase images of the upper abdomen, to include the whole liver and adrenals. These are possible sites of metastatic spread.

Incidental lung cancer findings require an urgent referral to the nearest rapid access lung cancer clinic/respiratory referral.

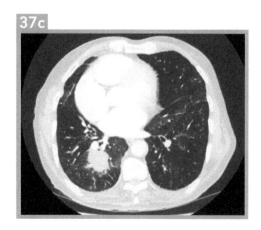

37c

# QUESTION 38

38  An 82-year-old male with a history of diabetes, rheumatoid arthritis and chronic
    kidney disease presents to the acute medical unit with symptoms of exertional
    breathlessness and peripheral oedema. There is no history of hypertension or
    ischaemic heart disease. He denies any chest pain and his troponin was negative.
    CXR showed evidence of bilateral costophrenic blunting. His ECG showed small
    complexes and a first-degree atrioventricular block. He is a lifelong nonsmoker and
    consumes alcohol in moderation. He claims that he had been referred recently to
    a national tertiary hospital for investigation of a heart problem. Among the battery
    of tests he has had are blood tests, cardiac biopsy, coronary angiography and a bone
    marrow biopsy.

i.    What echocardiographic features are present (38a, b)?

ii.   What could be the diagnosis?

iii.  What other echocardiographic features should be sought?

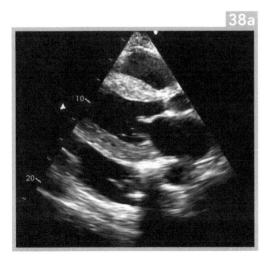
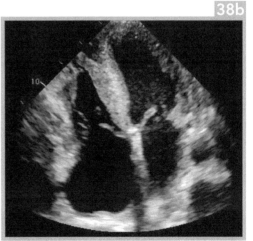

## Answer 38

**38i.** The arrows in 38c and 38d point at the thickened interventricular septum which has a 'speckled' appearance. The arrowhead in 38c points at a significant concomitant pleural effusion, likely due to heart failure. The ventricular wall hypertrophy is both concentric and biventricular and there is also a thickened interatrial septum.

**ii.** An infiltrative cardiomyopathy. Given the clinical history, amyloid heart disease is the most likely diagnosis. Senile cardiac amyloidosis is not an uncommon cause of restrictive cardiomyopathy in octogenarians. It results from deposition of amyloid fibrils in the myocardial interstitium. This condition is more common in males. Presentation with signs and symptoms of heart failure is the norm. There is no specific treatment available other than generic heart failure therapy.

**iii.** There is a fairly wide variety of echocardiographic findings associated with senile cardiac amyloidosis. There is an increase in left ventricular and/or right ventricular wall thickness which is almost always concentric, in the absence of a history of hypertension. The atria are both often dilated. There is usually an associated small pericardial effusion. There is a nonspecific thickened appearance of the valves and the interatrial septum. There may be a 'speckled' appearance of the myocardium but this is not pathognomonic of this condition as it is quite a common finding in other conditions such as hypertrophic cardiomyopathy as well as in other infiltrative cardiomyopathies. Left ventricular systolic function is often preserved initially and can progress to severe systolic dysfunction when the disease is advanced or end-staged. Diastolic dysfunction is almost inevitable with transmitral Doppler filling pattern often showing a restrictive pattern, which is due to raised left atrial filling pressures and decreased left ventricular compliance. No one single echocardiographic feature is diagnostic but a combination of several is useful in reaching a diagnosis.

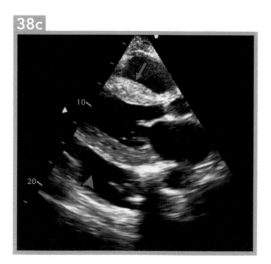

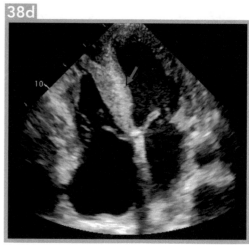

## QUESTION 39

39 A patient was noted to have a small right pleural effusion on CXR, after attending with a mild cough. CT was performed to investigate this (39a–d).

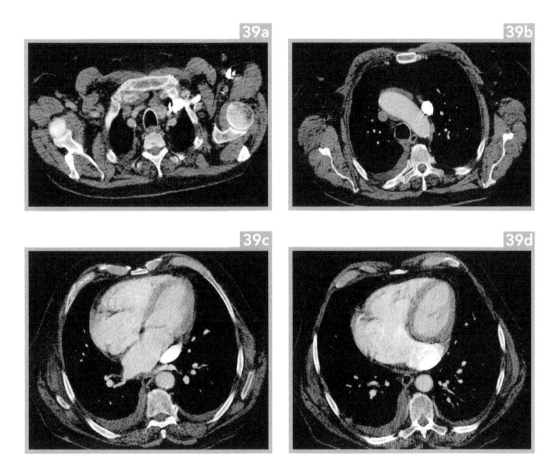

i.  What is the prevalence of this appearance in normal populations and in those with congenital heart disease?

ii. What features may cause clinical significance?

## Answer 39

**39i.** Axial CT images of the chest show a left-sided dominant but duplicate SVC, which drains into the main coronary sinus. This anatomical variant, found in 0.5% of the normal population but 5% of those with congenital heart disease, is generally an incidental finding but may be discovered after failed central venous catheter or pacing wire insertion.

The structures of the normal cardiac venous system are somewhat variable, but the coronary sinus is most consistent in its position. This runs along the inferior aspect of the heart in the arteriovenous groove before emptying into the RA.

The first branch of the coronary sinus is the middle cardiac vein, which runs in the posterior interventricular groove from base to apex. The subsequent two branches are the posterior vein of the LV and the left marginal vein. Here the coronary sinus becomes the great cardiac vein, which runs in the left arteriovenous groove with the circumflex artery. The vessel continues as the anterior interventricular vein in the anterior interventricular groove, extending from the base toward the apex running with the left anterior descending artery.

**ii.** A less common variant (10%) of cases involves insertion into the LA, creating a right-to-left shunt but this is usually not large enough to cause symptoms of cyanosis.

# QUESTION 40

40 A 65-year-old female presents to her GP with progressively worsening chest pain on exertion. She is known to be diabetic and is found to have a slightly elevated blood pressure. She has no smoking history. Clinical examination is normal. She was referred to the rapid access chest pain clinic and it was decided that she ought to undergo a functional test. Unfortunately due to arthritis in her knees she was unable to manage an ETT and therefore a MIBI scan was performed.

i. How is this type of scan performed?

ii. What does the MIBI scan show (40)?

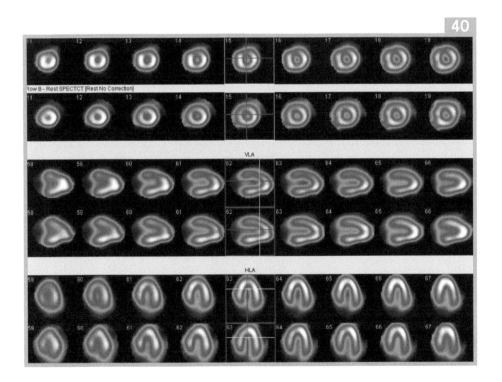

## Answer 40

**40i.** Technetium (99mTc) sestamibi is injected intravenously into a patient – this then distributes in the myocardium and its distribution is proportional to the myocardial blood flow. SPECT imaging of the heart is performed using a gamma camera to detect the gamma rays emitted by the technetium-99m as it decays. Two sets of images are acquired. For one set, 99mTc MIBI is injected while the patient is at rest and then the myocardium is imaged. In the second set, the patient is stressed either by exercising on a treadmill or pharmacologically (using dobutamine or adenosine stressors). The drug is injected at peak stress and then imaging is performed. The resulting two sets of images are compared with each other to distinguish ischaemic from infarcted areas of the myocardium.

**ii.** The short-axis scan images and the vertical long-axis scan images identify a difference in emission between stress (upper series) and rest (lower series). There is a defect in the anterior wall which is predominantly affecting the basal and mid left ventricular level segments which is present on the stress images but not on the rest images. Appearances are therefore of reversible anterior wall ischaemia consistent with a LAD territory stenosis.

# QUESTION 41

41  A 45-year-old male presents to his GP with shortness of breath. He has also noted swelling of his legs but did not report any episodes of chest pain. He is a lifelong nonsmoker with no previous history of diabetes or hypertension. Blood tests showed that he had a normal cholesterol and that his renal function was normal. On clinical examination he had elevated neck veins and had peripheral oedema. The GP referred the patient to a cardiologist who performed an echocardiogram. Poor echo windows made imaging difficult and the patient was referred for an MRI (41a–c).

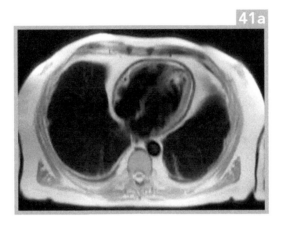

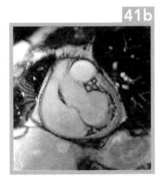 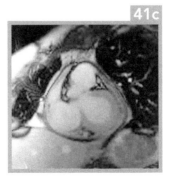

i.    What are the findings on the MRI?

**41i.** The axial and short-axis MRI images demonstrate circumferential pericardial thickening. The normal pericardial thickness is <2 mm but on these images it is shown to be ~5 mm. No obvious pericardial effusion is demonstrated. On the cine two-chamber images there is the classical appearance of a 'septal bounce'. The septal bounce is a paradoxical bouncing movement of the septum first towards and then away from the LV during early diastole (this is best assessed on short-axis cine MR images). The axial image shows some flattening of the left ventricular septum. Appearances are typical for constrictive pericarditis.

Constrictive pericarditis is a type of pericarditis which leads to diastolic dysfunction and potentially symptoms of right heart failure. Causes include:
● Infection – the most common cause being TB; viral infections; rheumatic fever.
● Sarcoidosis.
● Previous cardiac surgery.
● Radiotherapy.
● Chronic renal failure.
● Idiopathic.

Clinical presentation is dominated by restricted diastolic ventricular filling resulting in an increase in diastolic pressure in all four cardiac chambers. Patients typically present with symptoms of both left- and right-sided heart failure including dyspnoea, orthopnoea, easy fatiguability, hepatomegaly and ascites.

Constrictive pericarditis is characterised by fibrous or calcific thickening of the pericardium, which prevents normal diastolic filling of the heart. Calcification is usually seen along the diaphragmatic pericardium surrounding the ventricles. Tuberculous calcification is usually thick, confluent and irregular. In viral infections and uremia the calcification is thin. Calcification does not always imply constriction: only 30–50% patients show constrictive symptoms. CT is performed in many centres to determine the degree of calcification. CXR demonstrates pericardial calcification in 50% of cases.

It is important to remember that to diagnose constrictive pericarditis the patient should have symptoms of heart failure. Neither pericardial thickening nor calcification alone is diagnostic of constrictive pericarditis.

Differential diagnosis for the clinical presentation would include restrictive cardiomyopathy, e.g. due to amyloid. It is important to differentiate between constrictive pericarditis and restrictive cardiomyopathy. Both these conditions can show similar clinical manifestations and features of restricted ventricular filling on echocardiogram. MRI is very useful here for looking for infiltrative disease. Pericardial stripping is beneficial in constrictive pericarditis, but not in restrictive cardiomyopathy.

# QUESTION 42

42   A 63-year-old hypertensive male presents with tearing central chest pain, hypotension and absent right arm pulses. Images are obtained (42a, b).

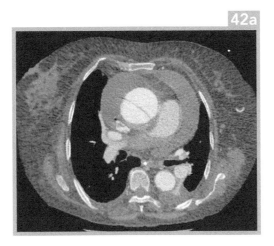

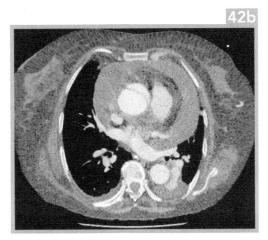

i.     What is the diagnosis and what complication is present?

ii.    What is the grading of this finding and what is the treatment for this?

## Answer 42

**42i.** Figures 42a and 42b are axial images from an arterial phase contrast enhanced CT of the chest. The images show an AP plane dissection flap within the aneurysmal ascending aorta, which is of a Stanford Type A. This is associated with a large pericardial effusion and small left pleural effusion, probably representing haematoma, which is suggestive of rupture into the pericardial sac. On CT, a Hounsfield attenuation of ~35–70 HU suggests a haemothorax/haemopericardium.

Aortic dissections are the generation of a vascular channel within the wall of the artery, caused by the separation of the intimal layer from the adventitia by circulating blood. They classically occur in fusiform aneurysmal aortas and are due to medial cystic degeneration of the cohesive medial layer of the artery. This creates a false lumen, which is often of larger calibre then the true lumen.

Aortic dissections most commonly present with sharp, tearing central chest pain, radiating to the neck and back and are often associated with murmur/bruit and peripheral pulse disturbance, such as asymmetry or absence. If rupture occurs, the patient can rapidly become haemodynamically shocked and breathless. Signs of pericardial tamponade and pleural effusion can be missed within the presentation of haemodynamic shock. Risk factors include hypertension, aortic stenosis, inherited collagen vascular disorders (Marfan's and Ehlers–Danlos syndromes), trauma and pregnancy.

CT imaging protocols should include a noncontrast CT initially to assess for crescentic high-attenuation intramural haematoma within the false lumen and to identify displaced intimal atherosclerotic calcification. Subsequent contrast enhanced aortogram demonstrates the two lumens within the vessel and allows assessment of acute extravasation, extent of dissection and involvement of branch vessels. ECG gating can be used (though not done routinely) if there is concern about the ascending thoracic aorta, given its mobility.

**ii.** Several different methods of classification are used for the grading of aortic dissections including Stanford classification and DeBakey classification. Stanford classification is the most straightforward with Type A involving the ascending aorta, and arise proximal to the left subclavian artery. Treatment of Stanford type A is urgent surgical graft, preventing rupture and involvement of the aortic valve. Type B dissections arise distal to the left subclavian artery and may be treated medically with antihypertensive medication.

# QUESTION 43

43  A 73-year-old female presents to the cardiology clinic with progressive breathlessness over the preceding 6 months. She has a bioprosthetic AVR performed 6 years ago for severe aortic stenosis, atrial fibrillation and diabetes mellitus. After her AVR, she led an active life but her symptoms have increased significantly in the last few months. Clinically, she had a pansystolic murmur heard loudest in the apical region radiating to the axilla and a flow murmur in the aortic area. She had bibasal crackles with mild peripheral oedema. An echocardiogram was requested and this showed that her prosthetic aortic valve was functioning well but she had severe mixed mitral valve disease which had not been noted before. A coronary angiogram was subsequently requested to assess her coronary arteries, with the view to referral for mitral valve surgery.

i.   Figures 43a and 43b show fluoroscopic images obtained during the coronary angiogram. What structure is the arrow pointing to?

ii.  What is mitral annular calcification and what are the implications of having this condition?

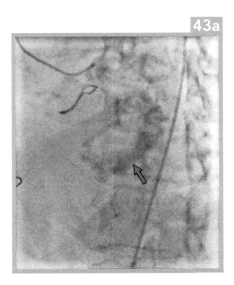
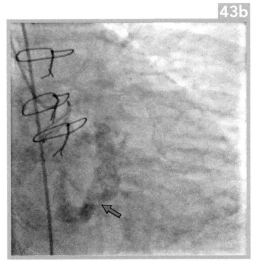

**43i.** The structure pointed to by the arrows is a ring of severe calcification of the mitral annulus seen in two different projections (left anterior oblique and right anterior oblique; 43c. d). The arrowhead is pointing to the bioprosthetic aortic valve. The sternal wires are visible on the left side of the image.

**ii.** Idiopathic MAC is a common finding with increasing age, with up to 10% of patients undergoing a transthoracic echocardiogram study found to have some degree of this phenomenon. Pathologically, MAC is characterised by degenerative calcification of the fibrous annulus of the mitral valve which occasionally extends into the subjacent myocardium. MAC is commoner in females, in older patients (especially over 65 years) and in patients with end-stage renal failure on dialysis. In the vast majority of cases, mild MAC is considered a benign incidental finding of no clinical significance. Patients with extensive calcification of the mitral annulus who require mitral valve surgery however, pose a major challenge to the surgeon and are at increased risk of surgery-related mortality and morbidity. Not uncommonly, the risk is deemed too high or the operation deemed technically not possible for the surgeon to proceed with mitral valve surgery (as is the case with this patient). A small but significant group of patients with extensive calcification may have conduction defects including atrioventricular block, which require pacemaker implantation. The pathophysiology in such patients is calcific infiltration of the conductive system. An unusual form of MAC is seen when there is an associated casseous necrosis (0.6% of all MAC), whereby there is an apparent mass most commonly in the posterior mitral annulus with a liquefied core. This apparent mass can be confused diagnostically with a tumour, thrombus or abscess. Often further clarification with other imaging modalities, such as multidetector CT and transoesophageal echocardiogram, is required to confirm or refute the differential diagnoses.

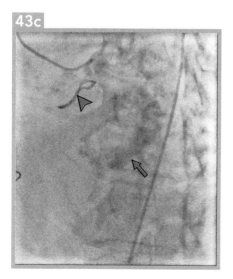

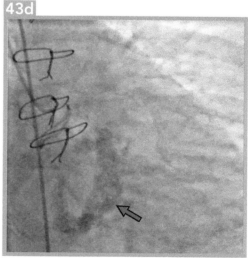

# QUESTION 44

44  A 56-year-old male presents to his GP with progressive shortness of breath. He is a lifelong smoker who has smoked ~30 cigarettes per day for 40 years. His shortness of breath is not related to exercise. He had had a single episode of haemoptysis. The GP sent him for a CXR which was abnormal and he was then urgently investigated further in the rapid access lung cancer clinic, where a mass lesion was identified on his CT chest.

i.  What is the important finding on the given images (44a–d)?

ii.  What are the common conditions causing this and what is the prognosis?

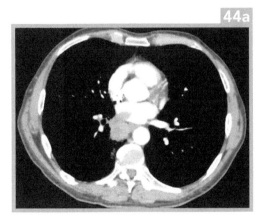

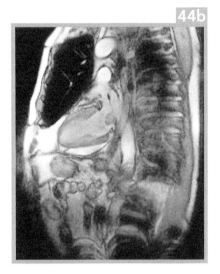

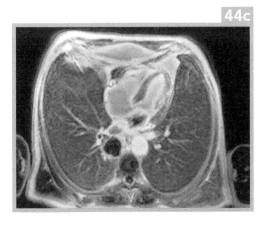

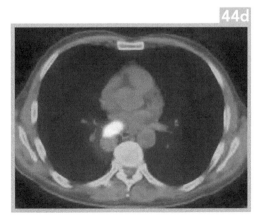

## Answer 44

**44i.** The CT (44a) demonstrates a mass lesion which is at the superior pole of the right hilum and appears to be invading the mediastinum. Soft tissue attenuation material appears to be within the superior pulmonary vein on the right and is extending into the LA. MRI images (44b, c) demonstrate more clearly the extension of the primary lung tumour via the pulmonary veins into the LA. In cases such as these it is sometimes difficult to determine whether the soft tissue material represents thrombus in the LA or tumour extension. The PET CT (44d) shows the abnormal tracer uptake in the LA and the right inferior pulmonary vein, which categorically confirms that this is tumour invasion.

**ii.** Soft tissue tumours which involve the pulmonary vein and the LA are most commonly due to an aggressive stage IV primary lung cancer or metastatic disease. Anatomically the LA is contiguous to the lung hilum, via the pulmonary vein. For this reason, direct invasion by lung cancer of an origin near the lung hilum is more likely to occur in the LA than in the RA. Tumour invasion usually occurs by one of two routes – either by growing along the pulmonary vein or by direct invasion of the posterior wall of the LA.

The other causes of LA soft tissue include: LA myxoma, LA thrombus, sarcoma, lymphoma and primary cardiac lymphoma.

The prognosis is very poor since this reflects a stage IV lung cancer. Thrombus can secondarily form on the surface of the invading soft tissue which can result in embolic events. Treatment at this stage is primarily mainly chemotherapy. In some cases where the invasion is limited to the posterior wall of the LA, a surgical resection of LA tumour along with pneumonectomy is attempted.

CT is the common modality of imaging to assess the extent of invasion of the posterior wall. Echocardiogram is more useful to know the direct extension through pulmonary veins in the case of primary hilar tumours. MRI and PET CT can also be of use in differentiating tumour and thrombus.

## QUESTION 45

45 A 70-year-old male presents with severe chest pain, positive troponin and ST segment elevation on ECG. A CMR was requested to determine viability. An adenosine stress perfusion image (45a), a rest perfusion image (45b), and a late gadolinium image (45c) are shown.

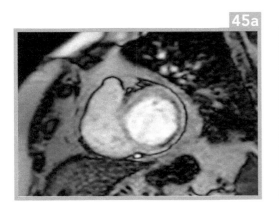

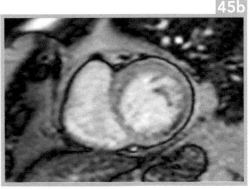

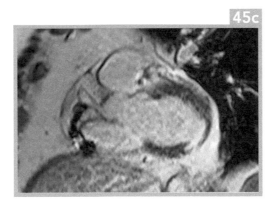

i. Describe the findings.

ii. Would this patient benefit from coronary revascularisation?

## Answer 45

**45i.** The stress perfusion image shows basal subendocardial hypoperfusion in the anterolateral and inferolateral segments. Figure 45b is a rest perfusion image showing a fixed perfusion defect in the basal inferolateral wall. The late gadolinium enhancement image (45c) shows subendocardial enhancement in the inferolateral wall. There is no thinning of the lateral wall. Appearances are consistent with an infarct in the circumflex territory, with the territory considered to be viable. There is also evidence of reversible ischaemia in this territory.

**ii.** Yes, the patient would benefit from revascularisation. The infarct is considered to be viable as there is less than 50% transmural gadolinium enhancement, indicating a high likelihood of functional recovery. The left ventricular wall is not particularly thinned and measures >5 mm in thickness. In addition, there is evidence of reversible ischaemia.

## QUESTION 46

46 A 63-year-old female presents to her GP with angina-like chest pain which is brought on by moderate exercise. She has no previous cardiac history. She is a nonsmoker with no history of diabetes, hypertension or hypercholesterolemia. She has no relevant past medical history and is on no current medications. Initial investigations revealed LBBB but no old ECGs were available for comparison. Normal CK and troponin T were found. Given the patient's low TIMI risk score, she was referred for a cardiac CT.

i.  What does the cardiac CT show (46a–c)?

ii. What medical management is used to optimise cardiac CT scans and what are the contraindications to these?

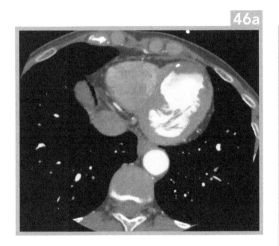

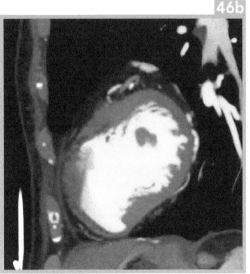

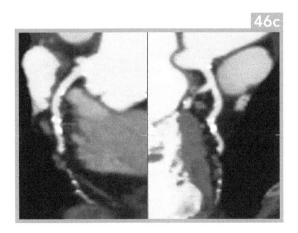

## Answer 46

**46i.** There are two images of the LV, an axial image (46a) and a sagittal reconstructed image (46b). These demonstrate focal thinning of the LV wall in the anterior, septal, lateral and inferior walls at the apical level as well as in the apex itself. These segments are also poorly enhancing compared to the rest of the myocardium. In addition there is a tiny focus of calcification seen within the wall at the apical septal segment. These appearances are consistent with a previous LAD territory infarct. As well as the infarct there is wall adherent, nonenhancing thrombus at the LV apex.

Analysis of the coronary arteries was performed (46c, oblique reformat) and this demonstrates a chronic occlusion to the mid LAD with minimal proximal disease.

**ii.** At the time of having a cardiac CT the scan quality is optimised by using beta-blockers and GTN. Beta-blockers are usually administered IV when the patient is on the table with metoprolol being the most commonly used agent. Reduction in cardiac motion leads to image quality improvement, so certainly achieving a lower heart rate results in better quality images, and a heart rate of below 60 beats per minute is the ideal. Following IV administration of metoprolol, the half-life of the distribution phase is approximately 10–12 minutes – allowing time for scan set up.

Beta-blockers are contraindicated in patients with:
- Asthma.
- Sinus bradycardia.
- Hypotension: blood pressure <90 mmHg systolic.
- Overt heart failure.
- Cardiogenic shock.
- Aortic stenosis.
- Second or third degree block.
- Right ventricular failure secondary to pulmonary hypertension.

If adverse cardiovascular effects are observed, IV therapy should be stopped immediately and the patient observed:
- Bradycardia and hypotension: atropine 0.5–1 mg initially should be given IV which can be repeated every 3–5 minutes up to a maximum dose of 3 mg.
- Hypoglycaemia: glucagon (1–10 mg) can be administered.
- Bronchospasm: salbutamol inhaler.
- Cardiac failure: IV frusemide 20–40 mg.

# QUESTION 47

**47** A 52-year-old male with a previous anterior MI was admitted to hospital following an out-of-hospital cardiac arrest from which he was successfully resuscitated. A 12-lead ECG revealed ST elevation in the anterior chest leads, but the ST elevation had been noted on an ECG performed 18 months previously. There was no antecedent history of chest pain on this occasion according to his wife. The patient had in-patient coronary angiography.

**i.** What do the fluoroscopic images show (47a, b)?

**ii.** What is the cause for this radiographic finding and what are the potential sequelae?

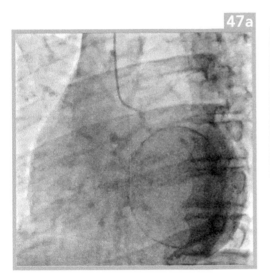

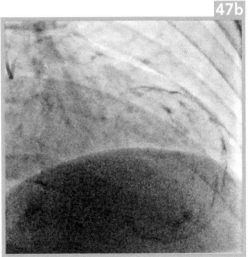

## Answer 47

**47i.** The fluoroscopic images show a calcified spherical structure overlying the cardiac silhouette. This is a calcified LV aneurysm.

**ii.** LV aneurysm is a potential complication from large MI resulting in transmural myocardial necrosis. While its overall incidence is low, it is most commonly associated with complete LAD territory infarct due to the large area of myocardium subtended by the LAD. The incidence of LV aneurysm complicating ST elevation MI has decreased over the years, mainly due to the changes in the management of these patients from thrombolytic therapy to primary percutaneous coronary intervention. A significant proportion of LV aneurysms contain mural thrombus that can potentially embolise. As such, patients with LV aneurysm can present with embolic symptoms such as transient ischaemic attack/stroke, bowel infarction, acute peripheral arterial occlusion and acute renal failure due to renal infarction, amongst others. Anticoagulation to reduce the risk of systemic embolisation is often recommended, especially if thrombus has been demonstrated within the aneurysm. Another potential sequela resulting from a LV aneurysm is the development of life-threatening arrhythmia. In such cases, aneurysectomy may be indicated to remove the aneurysmal sac, especially if medical therapy alone has failed to suppress ventricular tachyarrhythmia. The surgical removal of the aneurysm can also help improve the overall LV ejection fraction postsurgery, due to the removal of 'dead space' within the LV. There is about a 4% risk of rupture of LV aneurysm in the long term.

# QUESTION 48

48   A 59-year-old male presents to the accident and emergency department with worsening shortness of breath. There is a past medical history of atrial fibrillation, hypertension and heart failure. He has been feeling unwell with a mild pyrexia and his GP was treating him for a chest infection with antibiotics. Abnormal echocardiographic findings led to further investigation with a cardiac CT (48a–c).

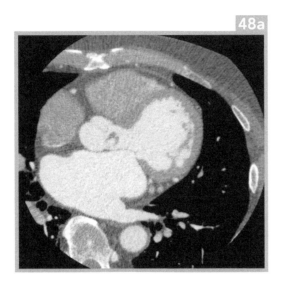

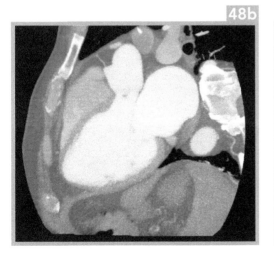

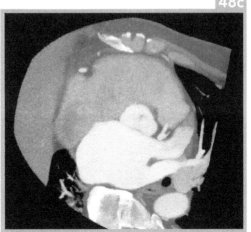

i.   What is the diagnosis?

ii.  What treatments are available for this condition?

**48i.** The cardiac CT demonstrates a focal ~7 mm soft tissue attenuation lesion related to the posterior valve leaflets. This tissue is nonenhancing, and given the clinical history is consistent with vegetations in a patient with bacterial endocarditis. Diagnosis should be confirmed with blood cultures. The patient failed to respond to antibiotic treatment and deteriorated with worsening heart failure. He was therefore referred for an AVR. Given the inherent risks of doing an invasive angiogram on a patient with endocarditic vegetations, a cardiac CT was performed. The patient had no evidence of coronary artery disease.

Typically, patients with endocarditis will present with a pyrexia of unknown origin but as the disease progresses the patients can develop symptoms of heart failure, shortness of breath, chest pain and embolic events. Individuals at an increased risk of developing endocarditis are those with predisposing factors:
- Rheumatic heart disease.
- Mitral valve prolapsed with mitral regurgitation.
- Previous endocarditis.
- Intravenous drug user.
- Bicuspid aortic valve.
- Prosthetic valve.
- Congenital heart disease.

**ii.** Treatment is usually with intensive IV antibiotic treatment for a minimum of 2 weeks. If, however, there is a failure to respond, then surgical treatment may be required. Indications for valve surgery due to endocarditis include:
- Heart failure.
- Uncontrolled infection.
- Significant valve dysfunction.
- Artificial valve infection.
- Extension of the infection into the heart (abscess formation).
- Recurrent emboli.

## QUESTION 49

49 A 25-year-old male is admitted to hospital with a 4-month history of abdominal and leg swelling coinciding with a gradual decline in exercise tolerance; he also describes symptoms of orthopnoea and paroxysmal nocturnal dyspnoea. There is no significant medical history. He is not on any regular medications and denies any illicit drug use and does not drink alcohol. He recalls two paternal cousins who died in their 30s with 'heart problems'. His ECG showed that he is in sinus tachycardia with a rate of 110 bpm and a LBBB. His chest radiograph showed cardiomegaly and evidence of pulmonary oedema. Routine blood test results were all normal. An echocardiogram was requested to assess his LV systolic function (49a, b).

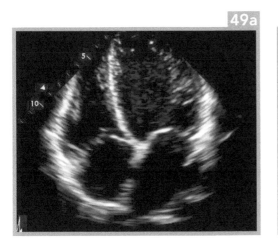
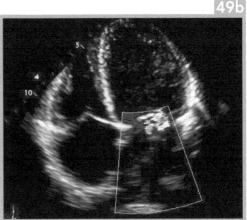

i.    What is the echocardiographic diagnosis?

ii.   How important is family history in this condition?

iii.  What tests should be performed to rule out a secondary cause of this condition?

## Answer 49

**49i.** Figure 49a, acquired in the apical four-chamber view, shows that all heart chambers are dilated with overall globular appearance of the heart. The interventricular septum and the ventricular walls are all thinned. There is evidence of a central jet of functional mitral regurgitation which results from mitral annular dilatation causing incomplete coaptation of the leaflet tips (49b). The patient's LV systolic function was confirmed to be severely impaired with an ejection fraction of 15%. It is unusual for a young patient to have these features on echocardiography. In the absence of precipitating causes, such as alcohol excess, long-standing systemic hypertension, viral myocarditis, chemotherapy-related cardiomyopathy, ischaemia/infarction and a number of rarer causes, this patient has idiopathic dilated cardiomyopathy.

**ii.** In about one-quarter to one-third of patients with idiopathic dilated cardiomyopathy, there is evidence for familial disease. Often the inheritance pattern that emerges from the family tree is that of an autosomal dominant inheritance. A number of X-linked diseases, such as Becker's and Duchenne's muscular dystrophy, are also known to cause dilated cardiomyopathy.

**iii.** All patients should have blood tests including renal function, liver function test, troponin, creatine kinase, erythrocyte sedimentation rate, ferritin, iron, transferrin, thyroid function test and viral serology. Coronary angiography should also be performed to exclude coronary artery disease as a cause of heart failure. In some patients, depending on their clinical history and presentation, additional blood tests that may be informative (not an exhaustive list) include red cell transketolase, selenium, carnitine, lactate, autoimmune antibodies and a viral screen (HIV, hepatitis B, hepatitis C). Occasionally, an endomyocardial biopsy can be useful. A cardiac MRI scan can identify patients with mid wall fibrosis, as evidenced by mid wall late gadolinium enhancement, an adverse prognostic indicator in patients with dilated cardiomyopathy.

## QUESTION 50

50  A 58-year-old male presents to the emergency department of his local hospital with chest pain. He has smoked 40 cigarettes per day for ~40 years and has a history of type 2 diabetes and poorly controlled hypertension. He describes a history of stable angina which has been medically controlled for the last 5 years. The patient says the chest pain he has presented with is different to his usual angina pain. Initial troponin T is negative. ECG shows LBBB but this is long-standing. The emergency department consultant requested a CT chest and selected images are shown (50a, b).

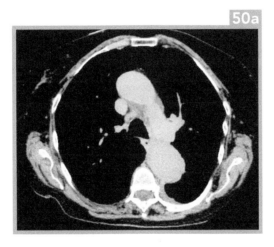

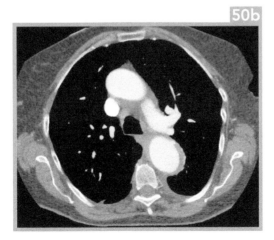

i.    What is the diagnosis?

ii.   What treatment options are available?

## Answer 50

**50i.** There are two axial images from a CT scan of the chest taken at the same level. Figure 50a is an uncontrasted image and Figure 50b is an arterial phase image at the same level. Figure 50b demonstrates a small penetrating aortic ulcer in the lateral wall of the proximal descending thoracic aorta. There is circumferential soft tissue around the lumen of the aorta which is less dense than contrast on the arterial phase scan, but is of relative high attenuation on the uncontrasted image; appearances would therefore be in keeping with intramural haematoma in the descending thoracic aorta.

Penetrating atherosclerotic ulcers of the thoracic aorta occur when atherosclerotic lesions rupture through the internal elastic lamina of the aortic wall. There is subsequent haematoma formation in the aortic wall between the media and adventitia. Penetrating atherosclerotic ulcer is typically seen in elderly individuals with a clinical history of hypertension and atherosclerosis and usually involves the descending thoracic aorta.

**ii.** There is still debate about what the best course of treatment is for these patients. There is a risk of disease progression to aortic dissection; development of a saccular aneurysm; and risk of spontaneous complete aortic rupture. Treatment of choice therefore is usually surgical with open repair and endovascular graft/stent insertion. In particular, persistent or recurrent pain, hemodynamic instability and a rapidly expanding aortic diameter have been considered indications for surgical treatment. Given that this is predominantly a disease of the elderly who are at significant risk at surgery, aggressive medical management and monitoring is also advocated.

## QUESTION 51

51 A patient with cough and mild SOB presented to the accident and emergency department, who arranged CXR which showed an abnormality. CT was requested to investigate this further, but correlation with previous cardiac MRI rendered this superfluous.

i. What are the features in the CXR (51a), CT (51b) and MRI (51c) which help determine the aetiology of this abnormality?

ii. What is the diagnosis?

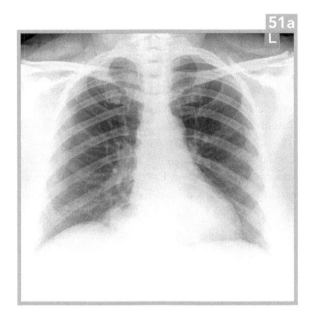

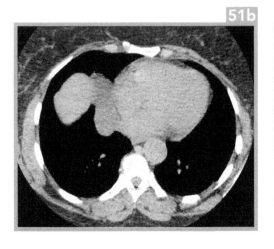

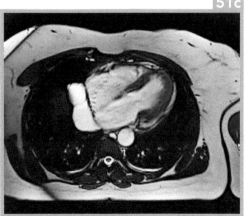

**51i.** The CXR shows a well-defined rounded lesion in the right cardiophrenic angle. No calcification or air fluid level is seen within it. The CT again demonstrates a well-defined lesion in the cardiophrenic angle with attenuation similar to that of water. On MRI the lesion is of high signal on T2 consistent with being fluid.

**ii.** Pericardial cysts are generally incidental findings but they have been rarely associated with chest pain and SOB, possibly due to vena cava obstruction. Classically, they appear in the cardiophrenic angle, most commonly on the right. Most are thought to be due to incomplete fascial development, although some have been reported in relation to pericarditis.

The main differential diagnoses for paracardiac masses are pericardial cysts, pericardial fat pads, LV aneurysms, sequestration cysts and diaphragmatic hernia. The density should be similar to that of water, although hyperattenuating cysts have been reported. Hypoattenuating paracardiac masses are most probably fat pads but dermoid cysts could have similar features. Rarely, in both pericardial and sequestration cysts, a thin rim of calcification is identified but this is never as thick as that seen in calcified LV aneurysms.

On MRI, pericardial cysts are low signal on T1, high signal on T2 and should not enhance, unless secondarily infected. Fat pads show high signal on T1 and T2 and also fail to enhance. Sequestration cysts have varying signal characteristics on MRI but are invariably high signal on T2.

LV aneurysms have a distinct appearance – see Question 72.

# QUESTION 52

52 A 78-year-old female had a chest radiograph performed because of a productive cough. She did not have any significant past medical history other than hypertension, for which she is on amlodipine and ramipril. Her CXR (52a) showed a prominent aortic knuckle which was not noted on a previous radiograph performed 2 years earlier. She was referred for a CT thorax with contrast to further evaluate this abnormality.

i. What does the CT image show (52b)?

ii. What is the usual presentation of patients with this condition?

iii. What are the indications for treatment?

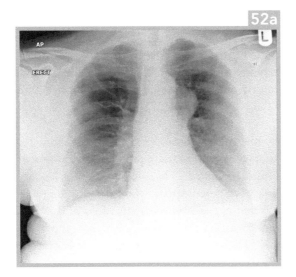

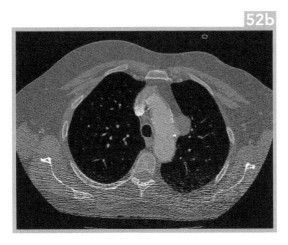

**52i.** The CT image shows a saccular aneurysm arising from the lateral aspect of the aortic arch (it measured 34 mm) beyond the origin of the left subclavian artery (52c, arrow). There is significant thrombus seen within the aneurysmal sac.

**ii.** Thoracic aortic aneurysm are often found incidentally, as patients are generally asymptomatic and CXRs are performed so widely that these aneurysms are often picked up before they are large enough to cause compressive symptoms. However, the discovery of a large aneurysm for the first time is not uncommon. A large ascending aortic aneurysm may cause aortic regurgitation with a wide pulse pressure and/or a diastolic murmur. Occasionally, an ascending aortic aneurysm can compress the superior vena cava, causing obstruction which would manifest as distended neck veins. Aortic arch aneurysm may cause traction on the recurrent laryngeal nerve resulting in hoarseness. Descending thoracic aneurysms can cause compression of the trachea or bronchus causing a wheeze, dyspnoea or cough. If the oesophagus is compressed then dysphagia may follow. Depending on the exact location of the thoracic aortic aneurysm, clots that are formed, especially within a saccular aneurysm, may embolise distally to cause ischaemia and/or infarction. This may involve the circulation to the limbs, brain, kidneys or viscera. Patients with connective tissue disorder such as Marfan's syndrome are at increased risk of accelerated aneurysmal formation and subsequent rupture.

**iii.** The risk of aneurysmal rupture is proportional to the diameter of the aneurysm. In general, elective repair of a thoracic aneurysm is recommended when the diameter of the aneurysm measures 5.5 cm. This measurement is less for patients with Marfan's syndrome and surgery is offered earlier when the diameter approaches 4.5 cm. Accelerated growth rate of the aneurysm regardless of the underlying aetiology is also an indication for earlier intervention. Patients who are undergoing aortic valve replacement should also have concomitant aortic root surgery if they have an aneurysmal aortic root (5 cm or larger).

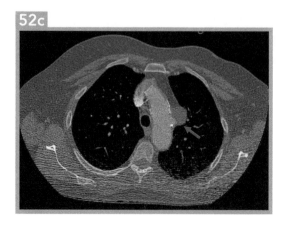

52c

# QUESTION 53

53  A 48-year-old patient was admitted with troponin-positive chest pain and sudden-onset pulmonary oedema. Rapid resolution of chest pain but refractory pulmonary oedema causing significant symptoms persists over the next few years. MPI showed normal LV resting uptake and function after initial presentation. Repeat MPI 12 months later showed similar uptake but moderately dilated LV and mildly reduced LV ejection fraction. CMR was performed to investigate this change in LV function.

i.  What are the imaging findings (53a, b)?

ii. What is the likely cause of the mitral regurgitation in this instance?

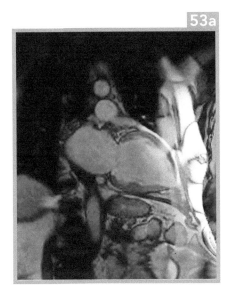

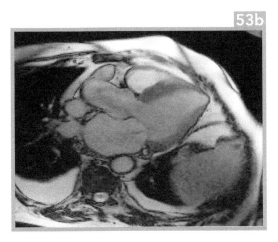

**53i.** Figure 53a is a two-chamber view which demonstrates enlargement of the LA and LV. Figure 53b is a three-chamber view and this demonstrates a visible jet seen at the level of the mitral valve. Appearances are therefore indicative of LA enlargement secondary to mitral regurgitation. The main causes for a dilated LA are: mitral valve disease (classically more so with stenosis); hyperdynamic shunts, such as PDA and VSD; and LV dilatation.

**ii.** Given the history of acute pulmonary oedema, with minimal LV dysfunction and absent uptake deficit on the first MPI, acute mitral regurgitation is likely, most probably secondary to chordae tendinae rupture or papillary muscle dysfunction.

The rapid development of LV dilatation over the course of 12 months without interim ischaemia is suggestive of significant mitral regurgitation, causing diastolic LV dysfunction.

CMR can show perfusion uptake, giving similar information to MPI but also allows for visualisation of ventricular motion and cine flow studies to assess valve pathology. In the above images, diastolically dilated LA and LV are associated with a clearly seen jet of dephased flow through the mitral valve in systole. Comparison between LV and RV stroke volumes allows an estimation of volume of regurgitation.

# QUESTION 54

**54** A patient has a history of lateral STEMI and a catheter angiogram was performed. There was a significant abnormality seen on the left ventriculogram. The patient developed worsening symptoms of LVF but poor images were obtained on TTE, so MRI was requested to assess function and viability.

**i.** What are the findings of the coronary angiogram (54a)?

**ii.** What is the abnormality on the left ventriculogram (54b, c)?

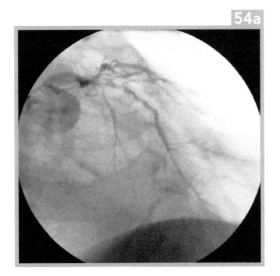

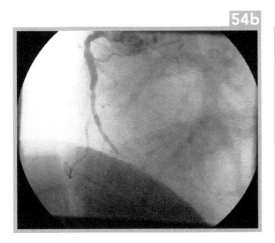

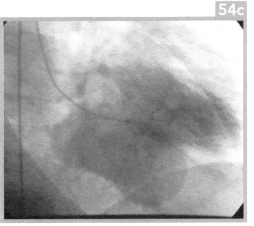

## Answer 54

**54i.** The invasive angiogram demonstrates long-segment disease within the circumflex artery which is unlikely to be amenable to angioplasty. There is a complete occlusion of the mid/distal RCA with a 6 mm long significant stenosis within the proximal aspect of the posterolateral branch.

**ii.** The ventriculograms show an outpouching from the inferolateral wall of the basal LV, consistent with a false LV aneurysm. Features that suggest this, as opposed to a true aneurysm, are: absent covering myocardium, position and morphology.

The MRI (54d–f) more clearly demonstrates the aneurysm which extends from the inferolateral wall of the LV. It appears to contain a significant amount of thrombus. The aneurysm has a relatively narrow neck with no visible myocardium in the wall of the aneurysm.

False aneurysms are essentially rupture of the LV myocardium, usually related to infarct but can be trauma related. The communication with the pericardium is limited by pericardial septations, but this still provides the classical morphology of a narrow neck at point of rupture and a larger blood- and thrombus-containing sac. The most common sites are the lateral wall, usually anteriorly.

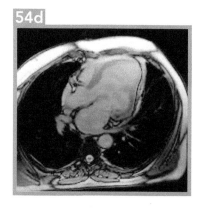
54d

Small aneurysms can be treated medically, using medications to reduce afterload, such as angiotensin-converting enzyme inhibitors. Embolic phenomenon may occur due to the thrombus within the aneurysm and this is an indication for cautious anticoagulation.

Surgical resection may be indicated if the LV aneurysm is causing LVF, embolic events or arrhythmias.

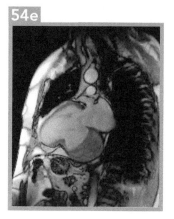
54e

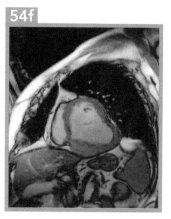
54f

## QUESTION 55

55   A 77-year-old male was admitted urgently to a district general hospital with severe breathlessness. He was confirmed to be in pulmonary oedema and was haemodynamically unstable. An urgent echocardiogram was performed in view of an ejection systolic murmur, and this confirmed critical aortic stenosis with a calculated aortic valve area of 0.5 cm². Left ventricular systolic function was mildly impaired. The patient was discussed with the nearest tertiary centre about in-patient urgent AVR. This was agreed upon but the patient's immediate transfer was complicated by the patient's haemodynamic instability and the on-call surgeon was about to begin a heart transplant at the surgical centre tying up resources in the next few hours. An urgent balloon aortic valvuloplasty was decided as a bridge to surgical AVR (55a).

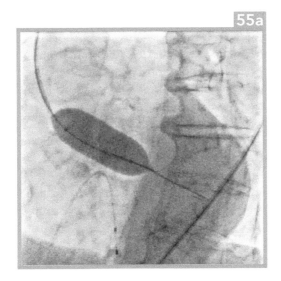

i.   What is balloon aortic valvuloplasty?

ii.  Why is balloon aortic valvuloplasty not more commonly performed?

iii. What are the current indications for balloon aortic valvuloplasty?

**55i.** Balloon aortic valvuloplasty is a percutaneous interventional procedure which involves the inflation of a suitably sized balloon across a stenotic aortic valve, thereby increasing the aortic orifice area. It is performed via a retrograde approach from the femoral artery. A guidewire is advanced up the aorta and across the stenosed aortic valve. This is then followed by inflation of the balloon which is positioned across the stenotic valve. In this patient, the aortic valve was ballooned with a 25 mm semicompliant (Cristal) balloon (55b, arrowhead) during rapid right ventricular pacing at 220 bpm; the temporary pacing wire can be seen positioned with the tip in the RV (55b, arrow). There was an immediate drop in transaortic gradient and the patient tolerated the procedure well with the help of opiates for analgesia. Postprocedural echocardiogram showed an increase in aortic valve area and no aortic regurgitation or pericardial effusion.

**ii.** Long-term data show that while balloon aortic valvuloplasty improved both aortic valve area and haemodynamic status in the short term, when compared to surgical AVR the results were inferior. The complication rates were also high, not least from access site bleeding (often femoral arterial site) due to the large size catheters required. Other common complications include stroke, other embolic complications and ventricular perforation. The restenosis rate is very high, estimated at about 80% at 15 months. Additionally, when compared to the natural history of patients with symptomatic aortic stenosis, balloon aortic valvuloplasty does not alter mortality to any significant effect.

**iii.** The ACC/AHA gives a Class IIb recommendation for balloon aortic valvuloplasty as a bridge to surgery in haemodynamically unstable patients with aortic stenosis. Additionally, there is also a Class IIb recommendation for the use of balloon aortic valvuloplasty as palliation for adults with severe aortic stenosis in whom AVR cannot be performed because of severe comorbid conditions.

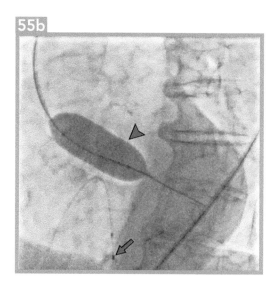

## QUESTION 56

**56** A 62-year-old male was referred to the cardiology clinic by his GP following a recent MI, now complaining of increasing shortness of breath on examination. TTE showed normal thickness of the LV but akinesia of the apical segments, associated with mild impairment of LV function. CMR was requested to assess myocardial viability for possible revascularisation (56a–d).

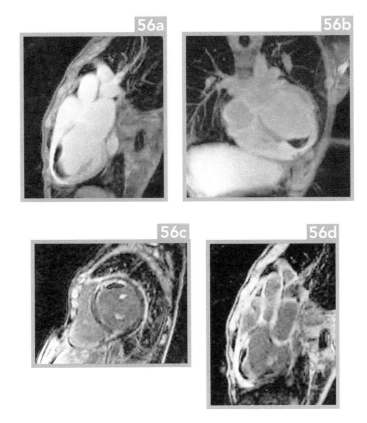

i.   Why is there apparent preservation of the wall thickness in this area on TTE?

ii.  What is the most likely common variant which may explain the finding on TTE?

**56i.** Figures 56a (three chamber) and 56b (four chamber) are early gadolinium images which are acquired as gadolinium is injected, such that there is contrast filling of the LV cavity. These images are often used to differentiate myocardium from thrombus. The images show a nonenhancing filling defect, adjacent to an area of thinned myocardium.

Figures 56c and 56d are late gadolinium images in which the myocardium is nulled (black) and which display transmural late gadolinium enhancement in the thinned myocardium. These features are consistent with an apical thrombus in the LV, associated with apical LV infarction.

Mural thrombi occur most commonly in relation to recent MI but are also seen in dilated cardiomyopathies and within LV mural aneurysms. The akinesia at the apex allows the formation of thrombus, creating an echogenic layer, adherent to myocardium. Small, immobile, layered thrombi of the apex are difficult to differentiate from myocardium on TTE, particularly when associated with slight aneurysmal dilatation. A clue to the presence of thrombus is an abnormally thickened apical myocardium.

**ii.** Normal variants can cause similar appearances on TTE and in the LV apex; the most common is an anomalous band, also known as false chordae. It can be difficult to distinguish myocardial tumours from more mobile and pedunculated thrombi. CMR is excellent in answering these diagnostic queries, demonstrating the akinesia, filling defect and noncontrast enhancement in thrombi and varied degree of contrast enhancement in cardiac tumours.

57   A 30-year-old male was referred to a cardiologist with symptoms of mild dyspnoea, fatigue and palpitations. A routine CXR showed cardiomegaly and his ECG showed RBBB. He also had a history of recurrent chest infections and a CT of the chest was performed (57).

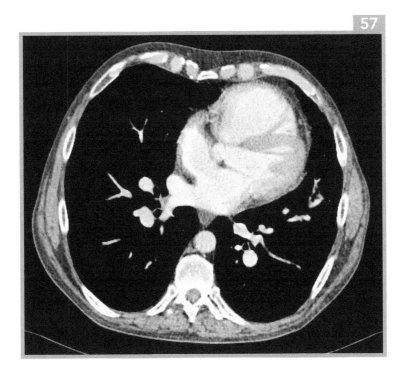

i.    What is the abnormality shown in the CT?

## Answer 57

**57i.** The single axial image of the chest shows a large defect in the interatrial septum at its superior portion (right atrial appendage is visible). Right ventricular enlargement can also be appreciated. Appearances would be consistent with an ASD and from the position, the most likely type is a sinus venosus defect.

ASDs represent approximately 10% of congenital cardiac defects and are the most common defect found in adults presenting over the age of 20 years. A sinus venosus defect is one type of ASD, accounting for ~5% of ASDs. Other ASDs include osteum secondum defects (70%), osteum primum (20%) and coronary sinus defects (<1%).

The sinus venosus defect is also called usual type and occurs in the superior portion of the atrial septum and is continuous with the SVC. The lesion is usually cranial and posterior to the fossa ovalis and is separate from it. It is usually associated with anomalous pulmonary venous drainage of the right upper pulmonary vein into the SVC. Rarely the defect is at the junction of the RA and IVC and is associated with anomalous connection of the right lower pulmonary vein to the IVC. The sinus venosus defects can also occur posterior to the fossa ovalis without bordering the SVC or IVC. These defects result in a left-to-right shunt through the defect.

The sinus venosus defects are present at birth; however, the clinical presentation depends on the size of the left-to-right shunt. During infancy and early childhood, they are usually asymptomatic.

The clinical symptoms depend on the size of the defect and the degree of left-to-right shunt. Easy fatiguability and breathlessness occurs in 60% of asymptomatic patients. Other symptoms include arrhythmias, dyspnoea and decrease in exercise tolerance test. These patients are usually diagnosed after discovering a murmur, fixed splitting of the second heart sound and right heart enlargement on ECG.

## QUESTION 58

58   A 56-year-old male was referred by his GP to the cardiology clinic with symptoms of breathlessness, palpitations and a new diagnosis of AF. The patient had noted that his symptoms have been gradually getting more pronounced over the last 5 months. He had been well otherwise, although he recalls being told when he was in his twenties that he had a heart murmur following a routine medical check. He was reassured at the time that this was an 'innocent' murmur. He is aware of two paternal cousins who had valve replacements in their fifties but does not know the details. On examination in clinic, he had a loud pansystolic murmur. He was referred for an echocardiogram (58a, b).

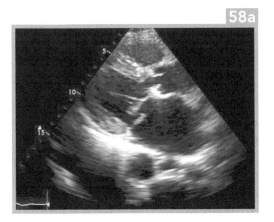
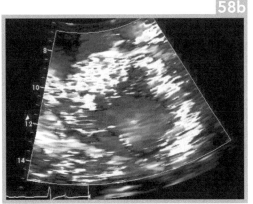

i.    What do the echocardiographic images show?

ii.   Is this condition unique to the mitral valve?

iii.   What is the natural history of this condition?

## Answer 58

**58i.** The parasternal long-axis image shows the prolapse of the posterior mitral valve leaflet (arrow, 58c) behind the plane of the mitral annulus during systole. The anterior mitral valve leaflet is positioned flushed with the annular plane. On colour flow Doppler, there is a large jet of mitral regurgitation (arrow, 58d) directed anteriorly 'hugging' the anterior atrial wall and extending all the way to the posterior wall. MVP is a condition that results from displacement of the mitral valve leaflet(s) into the LA, often accompanied by mitral regurgitation. Echocardiographically, MVP is diagnosed when the leaflets are seen to prolapse 2 mm or more behind the mitral annulus plane. There is often a myxomatous appearance of the leaflets, i.e. thickening of the leaflet tips. There may be LA and/ or LV dilatation depending on the severity of the mitral regurgitation. Dilatation of the LA is linked with an increased risk of developing AF. The development of AF is in fact a clinical indicator that significant atrial dilatation has occurred. If mitral regurgitation is allowed to progress untreated, LV systolic impairment will ensue. This may lead to involvement of the right heart and consequent pulmonary hypertension.

**ii.** There may be multiple valve involvement with about 40% of patients with MVP also having tricuspid valve prolapse. Pulmonary and aortic valve involvement is less common. It is therefore important to assess all valves when MVP is detected echocardiographically.

**iii.** The natural history of MVP is variable, ranging from being a benign asymptomatic condition to a more serious condition with significant morbidity and mortality. Predictors of cardiovascular mortality in patients with MVP are moderate-severe mitral regurgitation and impaired LV systolic function (LVEF <50%). Potential sequelae of MVP other than mitral regurgitation include rupture of the chordae tendinae and endocarditis. Some studies have suggested an increased risk of embolic cerebral events in patients with MVP. Sudden arrhythmic death is a rare complication seen in patients with familial MVP.

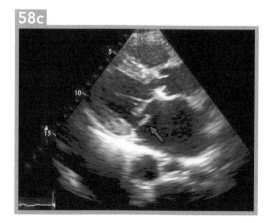

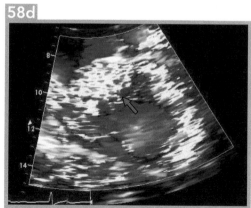

## QUESTION 59

59  A patient presents with a history of exertional dyspnoea over 12 months and several recent TIAs. A CXR shows mildly enlarged LA and pulmonary oedema. The ECG shows normal sinus rhythm. Transthoracic echo shows normal LV motion but a suspicious echogenic mass was seen in the LA (59a, b).

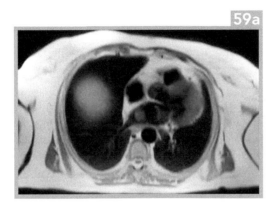

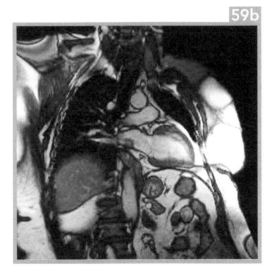

i.   What are the possible diagnoses?

ii.  How could you differentiate between them?

## Answer 59

**59i.** The images show a 2 cm filling defect attached to the posterior wall of the LA, on both 'black-blood' (HASTE – 59a) and 'white-blood' (fast steady state precision – 59b) images.

Possible diagnoses afforded by these images include left atrial thrombus and myxoma. The location is typical for thrombus, but although the fossa ovalis is the most common location for atrial myxoma, myxoma can also originate from this site. A layered appearance is typical for a thrombus and a pedunculated and mobile mass is more suggestive of a myxoma. Both are associated with embolic phenomenon but the presence of atrial fibrillation is more suggestive of thrombus.

Atrial myxoma is the most common of the cardiac tumours but these are rare tumours in general. Genetic prevalence is seen in Carney syndrome, which accounts for up to 7% of all atrial myxomas. Symptoms relate to obstruction at the mitral or tricuspid valve or to embolic phenomena. Emboli can result in systemic end–organ infarction or multiple chronic pulmonary emboli leading to pulmonary hypertension.

Atrial myxomas are also associated with Raynaud's phenomenon and digital clubbing, thought to be related to release of growth factors and inflammatory mediators, such as interleukin-6.

**ii.** Although the features listed above can suggest either thrombus or tumour, optimal differentiation can be achieved with gadolinium-enhanced MRI, showing definitive enhancement of the mass. This enhancement is clearly demonstrated on the four-chamber (59c) and two-chamber (59d) views. No imaging features can differentiate reliably between cardiac tumours, and definitive diagnosis is often only achieved on resection.

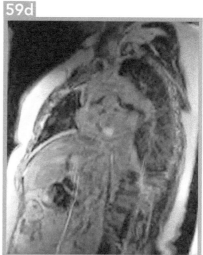

59d

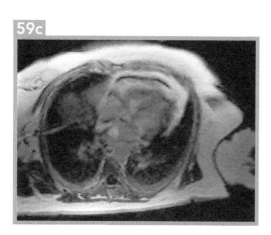

59c

## QUESTION 60

60 A 55-year-old female presents to the cardiologist with atypical chest pain. She is obese, but has no other known risk factors for coronary artery disease. She has no family history of heart disease. A radionuclide perfusion test was inconclusive due to the patient's body habitus. The patient went on to have a stress perfusion MRI for further evaluation (60a–d).

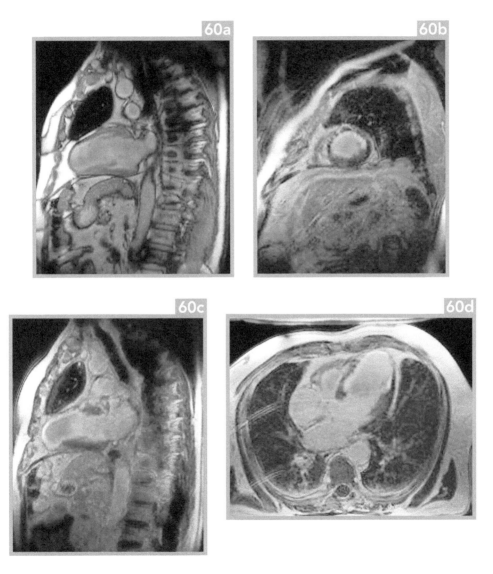

i.   What is the diagnosis?

ii.  Is the apex and anterior wall viable?

## Answer 60

**60i.** Figure 60a is a two-chamber cine MRI showing thinning of the anterior wall and apex of the LV (measured to be <5 mm). The subsequent images are short-axis (60b), two-chamber (60c) and four-chamber (60d) views with late gadolinium. The short-axis view shows subendocardial late enhancement of the basal anterior, anteroseptal and anterolateral segments. The two-chamber view shows transmural late enhancement of the anterior wall and apex of the LV. The four-chamber view demonstrates subendocardial late enhancement of the septum and lateral wall. The study indicates a LAD territory infarct.

**ii.** The myocardium at the apex and anterior wall shows transmural late enhancement and marked wall thinning and can be considered as nonviable. However, the septum and lateral wall show subendocardial late enhancement, no wall thinning and should be considered viable. The patient would benefit from revascularisation and functional improvement is expected. The patient should go on to have invasive coronary angiography.

# QUESTION 61

61 An on-call junior doctor was asked to review a CXR performed after implantation of a dual-chamber pacemaker for complete heart block (61a). His cardiology experience was limited but he wondered whether the ventricular lead was displaced as it was not 'directed' to the apex, as he had seen before on previous patients' radiographs.

i.    What does the CXR show (61a)?

ii.   What is the rationale for this ventricular lead position?

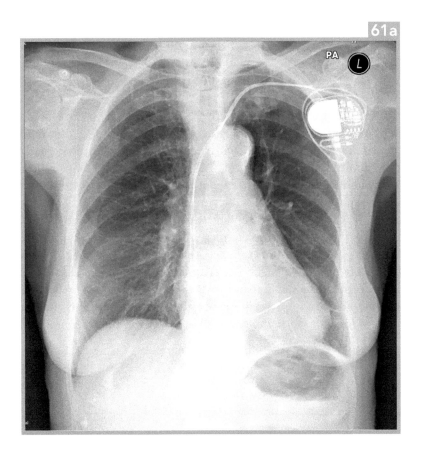

## Answer 61

**61i.** In Figure 61a the tip of the RV lead appears to be pointing in a 2 o'clock position (61b, arrow). This is the radiographic appearance of a mid RV septal pacing position, as opposed to RV apical pacing (the tip would point in a 4 or 5 o'clock direction). The junior doctor should check the implantation procedural notes to confirm that the operator has indeed chosen a mid RV septal position. There is no evidence of a pneumothorax. Figure 61c shows the corresponding lateral projection.

**ii.** Multiple studies have shown that chronic pacing of the RV apex for a bradyarrhythmia indication is associated with progressive heart failure over time and is also linked with a higher incidence of atrial fibrillation. In RV apical pacing, the impulse is conducted from the apex to the base of the heart, and from right to left ventricle, causing dyssynchronous ventricular activation and contraction, i.e. electrical and mechanical dyssynchrony. Alternative pacing sites within the RV have therefore been trialled to avoid or reduce these effects. Pacing sites such as the RVOT and high or mid RV septum have garnered significant interest because of the theoretical advantage of a more physiological ventricular activation, i.e. from base to apex, and from septum to the free walls. RV septal pacing is associated with a shorter duration of activation (as evidenced by shorter QRS duration), improved haemodynamics and less left ventricular remodelling. Selective-site pacing is technically more challenging and requires additional tools compared to apical pacing, including a septum-specific stylet to guide positioning of the ventricular lead on the septum and often a screw-in active lead is used to allow stable lead positioning. It is not surprising therefore, that one of the potential drawbacks of RV septal pacing is the difficulty in getting a stable septal position. Lead dislodgement postimplantation is hence a potential complication. With increasing operator experience and a much better understanding of the electrocardiographic data, fluoroscopic images and anatomy of the right ventricular septum/RVOT, increasing numbers of implanters are becoming more consistent and accurate in the placement of leads in the intended position higher up the interventricular septum.

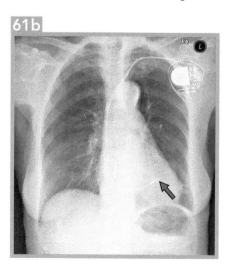

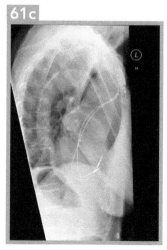

## QUESTION 62

**62** A 23-year-old patient presents for a follow up MRI having had a cardiac surgical procedure at 6 months of age.

**i.** What is the abnormality seen on the MRI (62)?

**ii.** What is the prognosis post procedure?

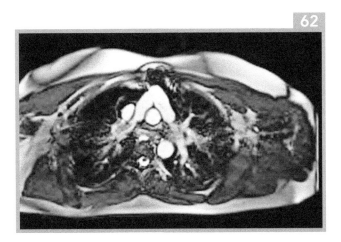

**62i.** The axial MRI image shows the pulmonary arterial trunk and the right and left pulmonary arteries bifurcating anterior to a posteriorly placed ascending thoracic aorta. This is the typical appearance of a patient who has undergone a previous arterial switch procedure (Lecompte procedure) for transposition of the great vessels.

TGA is a congenital cardiac anomaly presenting with cyanosis in newborn babies where the aorta originates from the RV and the pulmonary artery arises from the LV. This abnormality can be of two types:

- D-TGA – the atria and ventricles are in their normal position (AV concordance).
- L-TGA – there is inversion of the ventricles (AV discordance).

D-TGA (dexa-TGA) accounts for 10% of all congenital heart disease cases. It is a cyanotic congenital heart disease which is fatal without correction. There are two parallel circuits of blood – deoxygenated systemic circulation and an oxygenated pulmonary circulation. Mixture occurs due to a PDA or a VSD (in 50%). Symptoms can rapidly progress on closure of the ductus arteriosus. Surgical correction with switching of the position of the aorta and pulmonary trunk is performed with subsequent movement of the coronary arteries to the neoaortic root.

L-TGA ( leva-TGA) is a rare congenital cardiac anomaly. It is essentially congenitally corrected transposition of great arteries where the large vessels and ventricles are transpositioned and the RV is on the left side and LV on the right side (i.e. AV discordance and ventriculoarterial discordance). This is associated with other congenital cardiac anomalies such as VSD, pulmonary stenosis, tricuspid regurgitation and dextrocardia.

The direction of blood flow is as follows:
vena cava – RA – LV – pulmonary arteries – lung – pulmonary veins – LA – RV – aorta.

Isolated L-TGA is usually acyanotic and remains asymptomatic until adulthood. Patients can remain asymptomatic for life or else can then present with TR, right-sided heart failure, atrial arrhythmias and AV block. Symptomatology depends on the associated features, e.g. pulmonary hypertension if the left-sided AV valve is incompetent.

**ii.** Prognosis is usually excellent with a 5-year survival reported of up to 96%.

# QUESTION 63

63 A 1-month-old neonate presents with stridor and a failure to thrive. Images were obtained (63a, b).

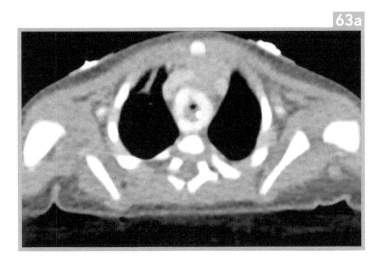

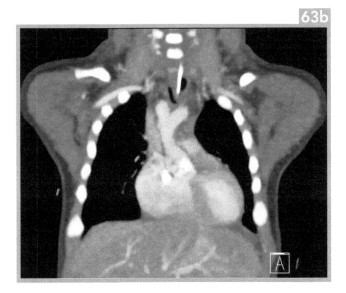

i. What is the diagnosis?

ii. How is this condition treated?

## Answer 63

**63i.** Axial (63a) and coronal reformatted (63b) images of an arterial phase CT scan of the chest are presented. The axial image shows a ring-like vascular structure which is surrounding the oesophagus and trachea (nasogastric tube is noted *in situ*). On the coronal image this can be better appreciated to be a double aortic arch.

Double aortic arch is the most common vascular ring anomaly of the aortic arch in which the two aortic arches form a complete vascular ring. This is caused by persistence of both fetal arches, i.e. the right and left IVth brachial arches. This is also the most symptomatic of all the vascular rings. It is however, rarely associated with other congenital cardiac anomalies.

The two arches join and form the descending thoracic aorta, which is usually left sided, but may however, sometimes be right sided or in the midline. In some cases the end of the smaller left arch closes and forms a fibrous cord, which can still give the symptoms of stridor and so on. The right arch is usually higher (75%) and supplies the right common carotid and right subclavian arteries. The left arch is usually lower and supplies the left common carotid and left subclavian arteries.

Patients usually present with symptoms of stridor, repeated apnoea, respiratory distress and dysphagia. Symptoms get worse after feeding and lead to a failure to gain weight. The symptoms may start at birth.

On CXR, there is evidence of soft tissue/vascular shadowing on both sides of the trachea, with the right arch higher and larger than the left arch. This gives the impression of a widened mediastinum. Barium swallow is often performed due to the symptoms of dysphagia and to exclude a tracheoesophageal fistula which can produce somewhat similar symptoms. This shows bilateral narrowing of the oesophagus at different levels due to indentation of the aorta on the oesophagus. On the lateral view there is posterior indentation of the oesophagus which is a nonspecific sign of a vascular ring. In neonates echocardiography allows images of the aorta and can show two separate aortic arches, with each arch giving a carotid and subclavian artery.

CT/MRI easily demonstrates the cross-sectional anatomy.

**ii.** Treatment is by thoracotomy with division of the smaller aortic arch. Some patients have persistent symptoms due to respiratory tract obstruction and compression. Prognosis depends on associated anomalies.

64   A 48-year-old female with recurrent TIAs was referred to the department of cardiac investigations for a bubble contrast study. She otherwise has no significant medical history. Her 12-lead ECG showed that she was in sinus rhythm. Her standard TTE study was reported as normal. The apical four-chamber view acquired as part of the TTE examination is shown (64a).

i.    What is a bubble contrast study?

ii.   Figure 64b was obtained with the patient in quiet respiration after the injection of agitated saline. What does it show?

iii.   The patient was asked to perform a Valsalva manoeuvre and Figure 64c was obtained just after the patient was asked to release/terminate the Valsalva manoeuvre. What does it show?

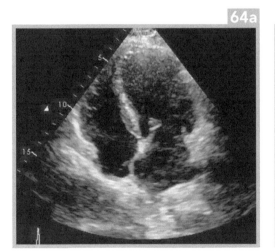

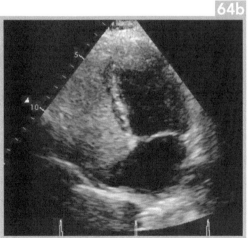

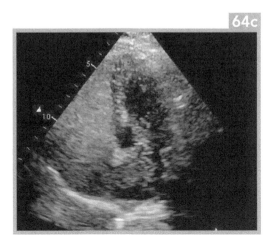

## Answer 64

**64i.** A bubble contrast study is an echocardiographic technique that uses a saline solution which is agitated by mixing it back and forth between two syringes, resulting in the production of suspended microbubbles. The agitated saline is then injected into the left antecubital vein and can be seen to pass into and opacifying the right heart. A bubble contrast study is used to identify atrial shunts and to confirm the presence of a PFO. Patients who have recurrent stroke symptoms in the absence of obvious risk factors, such as atrial fibrillation or carotid artery disease, should have a bubble contrast study to rule out a PFO. The presence of a PFO may cause paradoxical embolism of thrombi from the venous system into the arterial system via the PFO, resulting in recurrent embolic stroke.

**ii.** Figure 64b shows that the microbubbles have rapidly opacified the RA and RV. No opacification of the left heart is seen, indicating that there is no apparent right-to-left shunt in quiet respiration with all bubbles confined to the right heart. If there is a major shunt, e.g. large ASD, shunting may be evident even at rest (which is not the case here).

**iii.** As no bubbles appeared in the left heart, a repeat injection was performed with a Valsalva manoeuvre (64c, d). The crucial period of a Valsalva is when the patient relaxes, as it is then that the right-sided pressure transiently rises relative to the left. The appearance of bubbles in the left heart within five cardiac cycles following right heart opacification and release of Valsalva suggests an intracardiac shunt. In this patient, the arrow in 64d shows the bubbles crossing from the RA to the LA via the interatrial septum within two cardiac cycles, indicating the presence of a PFO. The PFO probably played a pathophysiological role in her recurrent TIA symptoms.

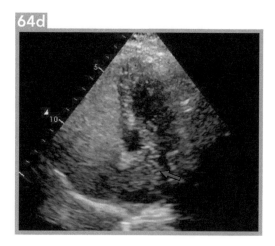

65 A 30-year-old female was admitted with chest pain. Troponin T was negative and the ECG was normal. She had no known risk factors for coronary artery disease, except for a family history of ischaemic heart disease. She underwent a cardiac CT with a low pretest probability of coronary artery disease. Images from the CT are shown (65a–c).

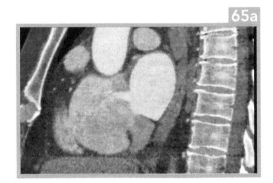

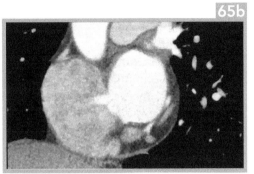

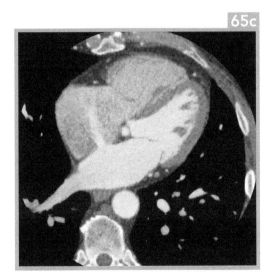

i.   What is the diagnosis?

ii.  Are patients usually symptomatic?

## Answer 65

**65i.** The CT shows a jet of contrast arising from the LA (the density of the contrast is the same as that in the LA) going towards the RA. The diagnosis in this case was PFO.

To understand the development of a PFO, it is helpful to be familiar with the embryology of the heart. The primitive atrium is divided into two by the septum primum which grows from the roof of the atrium towards the endocardial cushions. Before the fusion is complete, a defect appears in the superior part of the septum, termed the foramen secundum. A second membrane, the septum secundum then grows to the right of the septum primum. This is never complete and has a free lower edge which, however, extends low enough to overlap the foramen secundum and hence to close it. These two overlapping defects in the septa form the foramen ovale which shunts blood from the right to the left side of the heart in the fetus, allowing blood to bypass the nonfunctional fetal lungs.

After birth, the pressure in the pulmonary circulatory system drops, thus causing the foramen ovale to close. If this opening fails to close naturally soon after the baby is born, the hole is called a PFO.

**ii.** No – patients with PFO are usually asymptomatic. PFO occurs in approximately 25% of adults and are usually of little haemodynamic consequence. PFOs have the potential of right-to-left shunt and have been linked to paradoxical thromboembolic stroke. Patients may have a history of stroke or TIA of unexplained aetiology. PFO has also been linked to symptoms of migraine and decompression sickness.

A PFO can be detectable with echocardiography. If a PFO is an incidental finding, the patient will not require any treatment. There is debate as to whether patients experiencing stroke or TIA require anticoagulation therapy or closure of the PFO (either surgical or percutaneously).

## QUESTION 66

**66** A 30-year-old male, with increasing SOB on exercise, presents as an emergency after an episode of exertional syncope. On clinical examination there was a loud systolic murmur on auscultation. There was no evidence of hypertension.

**i.** What are the two likely diagnoses, given the history? Why can only one of these explain the features in images 66a–c?

**ii.** What pattern of late gadolinium is typical in this condition?

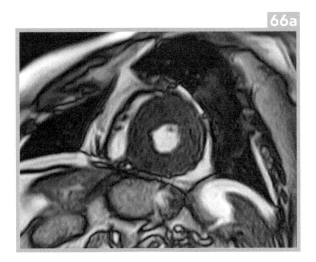

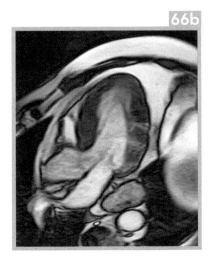

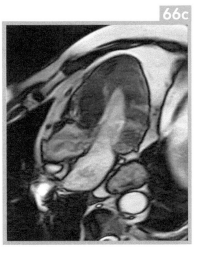

## Answer 66

**66i.** The symptoms and signs are of LVOT obstruction and the differential is of aortic stenosis or HOCM.

The imaging shows a nondilated hypertrophied LV myocardium, which, in the absence of a cause, such as longstanding hypertension, is indicative of HOCM. There is dynamic narrowing of the LVOT in systole, with anterior motion of the mitral valve leaflet towards the septum (66c). This is diagnostic of HOCM.

Diagnosis of HOCM is usually made on echocardiography or cardiac MRI. Measurement of diastolic wall thickening, such that the interventricular septum measures >13–14 mm; the posterolateral wall measures >11 mm; or the ratio of these being >1.3:1 is indicative of HOCM.

HOCM is a disease with a marked autosomal dominant genetic component but variable phenotypic penetrance. Imaging appearance and symptomatology depend on the remodelling and degree of hypertrophy which occur due to the underlying myocardial disarray. The disease can manifest throughout the LV (symmetric/concentric HOCM) or display asymmetric hypertrophy (asymmetric septal HOCM or apical HOCM). When basal in distribution and involving the septum this leads to subaortic stenosis and causes the classical HOCM pattern. The degree of stenosis is exacerbated by the anterior motion of the mitral valve, at least in part thought to be due to the Venturi effect of the higher velocity Vmax of the LVOT, with associated mitral regurgitation.

Increasing hypertrophy due to increasing obstruction leads to higher systolic pressures and worsening mitral regurgitation and resultant LA dilatation. This LA dilatation is associated with the development of AF, and further arrhythmogenesis occurs in areas of scarring within the hypertrophied segments.

**ii.** The fibrotic areas show late gadolinium enhancement, characteristically intramural, with sparing of the subendocardium.

# QUESTION 67

67 A 62-year-old male was brought into hospital following an out-of-hospital cardiac arrest. He was successfully resuscitated by the paramedics who managed to record a rhythm of ventricular tachycardia degenerating into ventricular fibrillation, prior to defibrillation. He had no risk factors for ischaemic heart disease and was otherwise fit and well. He proceeded to have coronary angiography which revealed smooth unobstructed coronary arteries. Echocardiography demonstrated normal left ventricular systolic function. Electrolytes were all within normal limits. His resting 12-lead ECG was also otherwise normal. He was referred for an ICD on the grounds of secondary prevention.

i. The postimplantation CXR is shown (67a: PA projection; 67b: lateral projection). What is the explanation for the lead positions?

ii. How common is this condition?

iii. What problems does it pose?

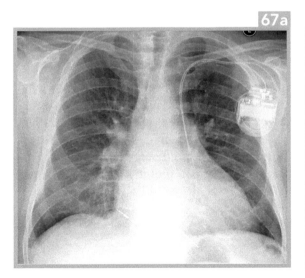
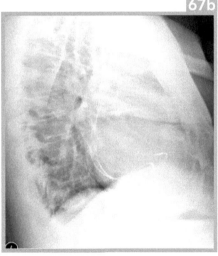

## Answer 67

**67i.** This patient has a persistent left-sided SVC giving rise to the appearance of both the atrial and ventricular leads positioned to the left of the spine. A left-sided SVC forms due to the failure of the anterior cardinal vein to obliterate during normal fetal development. The anterior cardinal vein subsequently develops into a persistent left-sided SVC which traverses anterior to the left hilum and joins either the coronary sinus in 90% of cases (which then drains into the RA) or the LA in 10% of cases. In the former scenario, the anatomical anomaly results in no functional significance, but in the latter it results in a right-to-left shunt. In the majority of patients with persistent left SVC (about 80%), the right-sided SVC is also present but often much smaller than the left.

**ii.** A left-sided SVC is the most common congenital venous anomaly in the thorax. It has a prevalence of about 1 in 250 in the general population and about 1 in 25 among patients with congenital heart disease. Most patients with an isolated persistent left-sided SVC are not aware that they have such an anomaly as the condition is not associated with symptoms, unless there is a large right-to-left shunt (i.e. SVC to LA shunt). In most patients, the condition is only discovered when a procedure or a scan is performed for other reasons, as is the case with this patient. When occurring in the presence of a congenital heart condition, the commonest associations are ASD, VSD, TOF, pulmonary stenosis and anomalous pulmonary venous return.

**iii.** Having a left-sided SVC poses a challenge to the operator performing a device implantation due to the 'awkward' anatomy, not least the acute angle between the coronary sinus os and the right ventricular inflow tract (as in this case). All of the tools that aid the implantation of a pacemaker or ICD are designed for a right-sided SVC. Often the operator has to improvise with different curvature of the stylets to try to place the lead tips in a stable position. Almost always, active screw-in leads are required to secure these positions so as to avoid lead dislodgement, which is not uncommon in these circumstances.

# QUESTION 68

68 A 48-year-old diabetic male presents to the chest pain clinic with atypical chest pain. On examination, he is hypertensive. A radionuclide perfusion scan was performed to assess for coronary artery disease, but was inconclusive. The patient therefore went on to have a stress perfusion MRI (68a is the adenosine stress perfusion image, 68b is the rest perfusion image).

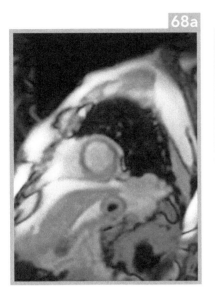
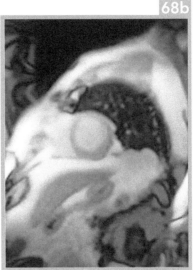

i.    What is the diagnosis?

ii.   Would the patient benefit from coronary revascularisation?

**68i.** The adenosine stress image demonstrates subendocardial nonenhancement in the mid anteroseptal and inferoseptal segments. The rest perfusion image shows normal enhancement in the entire myocardium. The study is indicative of reversible ischaemia in LAD territory.

**ii.** Yes, the patient would benefit to go on to invasive coronary angiography.

Myocardial perfusion imaging is indicated in patients with known or suspected coronary artery disease. Radionuclide imaging is the most widely used modality for investigating myocardial perfusion. However, MRI is an alternative technique being increasingly used offering superior spatial resolution to scintigraphy and therefore is more accurate for identifying subendocardial perfusion defects. In addition, scintigraphy is subject to attenuation artifacts in high body mass index patients or patients with large breasts. MRI also offers the advantage of being free from ionising radiation.

The underlying principle of the test is that under resting conditions a significant stenosis of a coronary artery does not usually cause a decrease in myocardial perfusion. This is because the resistance distal to the stenosis reduces to maintain flow. However, under conditions of stress, arteries with significant stenosis receive less blood flow than normal arteries.

In stress perfusion MRI imaging, a pharmacological agent such as adenosine, dobutamine or dipyridamole is injected to induce 'stress'. Adenosine is the agent commonly used and is infused for at least 3 minutes at a rate of 140 µg/kg/min in order to induce maximal hyperaemia. Continuous heart rate and blood pressure recording is performed. During the last minute of adenosine infusion (at peak vasodilatation), an intravenous bolus of 0.05 mmol/kg gadolinium is injected to image the first-pass myocardial perfusion. Perfusion abnormalities appear as regions of myocardium with hypo- or nonenhancement.

A rest perfusion study can be performed to distinguish between a significant stenosis and prior myocardial infarction. The same scan protocol is performed without adenosine at least 10 minutes after the stress perfusion imaging. The presence of a perfusion defect at stress but not at rest is called an inducible perfusion defect and indicates reversible ischaemia and a significant stenosis. A perfusion defect present both at stress and rest is called a matched perfusion defect and indicates scar tissue likely from a previous infarction.

69 A 35-year-old female emigrating to Canada was required to have a CXR as part of her health screening (69a).

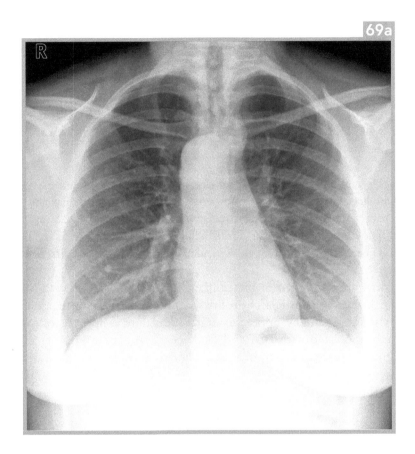

i. What is the abnormality?

ii. Is it associated with any cardiac abnormality?

## Answer 69

**69i.** The CXR shows an absence of an aortic knuckle from its usual position on the left and it can be seen in fact on the right; appearances would therefore be in keeping with a right-sided aortic arch. Selected images from an unenhanced chest CT (69b, c) are included which confirm a right-sided aortic arch. It is also worth noting on the CXR that the cardiac outline is normal with no evidence of cardiac enlargement. There are no features of heart failure in the lung parenchyma.

Figure 69c demonstrates the origins of the great vessels and the left and right common carotid artery origins are well visualised. In addition the left subclavian artery is seen arising as the final branch from the aortic arch, with the vessel seen passing behind the oesophagus. This is therefore a case of right aortic arch with aberrant left subclavian artery.

**ii.** Right aortic arch with aberrant left subclavian artery is the commonest type of right aortic arch anomaly and is the second commonest cause of a vascular ring after a double aortic arch. It is only rarely associated with congenital heart disease, i.e. in ~5% of cases. The commonest cardiac abnormalities it is associated with are TOF, ASD, VSD and coarctation. Usually it is an incidental finding in asymptomatic patients.

Right aortic arch with mirror image branching (left subclavian artery will be the first branch from the aortic arch) is the second commonest aortic arch abnormality. This is associated with cyanotic congenital heart disease in ~90% of cases. It is most commonly associated with TOF (~85% of cases), truncus arteriosus, transposition of the great vessels and tricuspid atresia. There is no vascular ring and no retro-oesophageal component.

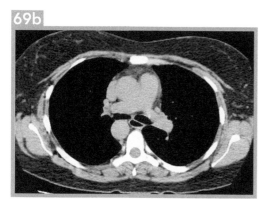

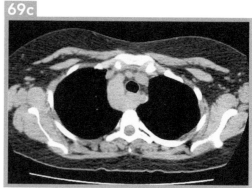

# QUESTION 70

70 A 39-year-old female, normally fit and well, presents to hospital with sudden-onset of severe chest pain radiating down her left arm. She is a nonsmoker and not on any prescribed medications. Clinical examination revealed pure heart sounds with no murmurs. Lung auscultation was unremarkable. Her 12-lead ECG confirmed inferior STEMI. She was loaded with dual antiplatelet therapy and was transferred to the catheterisation laboratory for coronary angiography.

i. What does the fluoroscopic image show (70a)?

ii. What is the cause of this condition?

iii. What is the treatment for this condition?

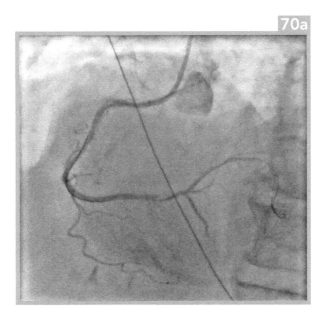

## Answer 70

**70i.** Figure 70a shows dissection of the distal right coronary artery (70b, arrow). This is the culprit lesion causing the inferior STEMI.

**ii.** Coronary dissection can occur spontaneously or as a result of coronary intervention, chest trauma or extension from aortic dissection. Dissection causes the separation of the layers of the arterial wall which is made of three layers – intima, media and adventitia – creating a false lumen. Spontaneous coronary artery dissection is very rare, with the majority of patients affected being women in their 30s. About one-third of cases occur in the peripartum period. Changes in the sex hormones during pregnancy, especially the high levels of oestrogen, are thought to alter the normal arterial wall architecture increasing the susceptibility of spontaneous dissection. In some cases, spontaneous coronary artery dissection occurs in patients with connective tissue disorder such as Marfan's syndrome and Ehlers–Danlos syndrome. Occasionally patients may present with a spontaneous coronary artery dissection as a first presentation of their undiagnosed connective tissue disorder.

**iii.** Primary percutaneous coronary intervention is the reperfusion strategy of choice if there is complete or significant luminal obstruction. In this patient, a stent was deployed at the area of dissection with restoration of normal blood flow (70c, arrow). Thrombolytic drug therapy is contraindicated because it can cause propagation of the dissection. There is a high mortality associated with peripartum spontaneous coronary artery dissection, estimated at 35–40%. A high proportion of patients with spontaneous coronary artery dissection have recurrent dissections, indicative of a general vessel structural weakness.

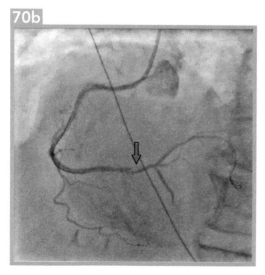

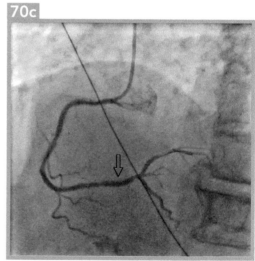

## QUESTION 71

71 A 56-year-old male was brought in by ambulance with central chest pain at rest, radiating to his jaw. He is a smoker with a 30-pack-year history. He is not on any regular medications. There is a strong family history of ischaemic heart disease. His ECG showed ST elevation in leads II, III and aVF. He was transferred to the catheterisation laboratory for emergent coronary angiography with the view to PCI.

i. What does the coronary angiogram show (71a)?

ii. What is the best treatment option for this patient?

iii. What are the potential complications of PCI?

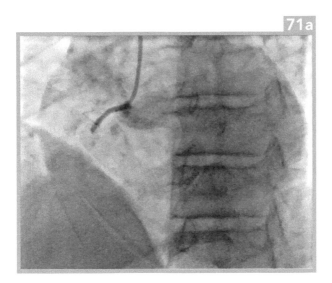

## Answer 71

**71i.** There is complete occlusion of the right coronary artery which has resulted in the patient's presentation with a STEMI (71b, arrow).

**ii.** As this patient has a complete occlusion of a coronary artery, primary angioplasty is the treatment strategy of choice. The final angiographic result shows no evidence of any luminal stenosis (71c). The mid right coronary artery was stented with a DES. The current consensus is that all patients with DES should be on dual antiplatelet therapy for 12 months (30 days for patients with bare metal stents). The risk of stent thrombosis is increased significantly in patients who prematurely discontinue dual antiplatelet therapy. Stent thrombosis is associated with a mortality rate of between 20% and 45%.

**iii.** The overall in-hospital mortality associated with PCI is less than 1% in elective PCI and as high as 2-4% in patients presenting with STEMI. Periprocedural myocardial infarction may occur and often in the context of acute artery closure, distal embolisation and no-reflow, side branch occlusion and acute stent thrombosis. In about 1 in 250 cases of patients undergoing PCI, emergency CABG is required. The incidence of PCI-related stroke is in the order of 0.2–0.3% and when this happens, the in-hospital mortality increases significantly to 25–30%. Vascular complications due to PCI are related mainly to vascular access. Common femoral vascular complications are access site haematoma, pseudoaneurysm, atrioventricular fistula, arterial dissection and retroperitoneal haemorrhage. Periprocedural use of glycoprotein IIb/IIIa inhibitors is associated with an increased risk of access site bleeding. Access site bleeding is reduced with a radial artery approach and increasingly these days, transradial PCI is now the default approach.

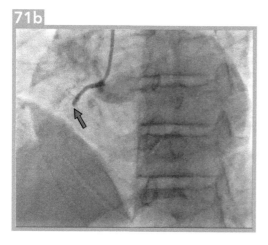

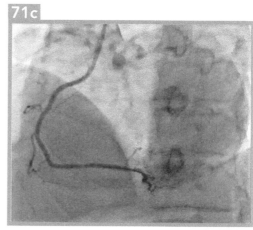

## QUESTION 72

**72** A 70-year-old female, with a history of previous myocardial infarction many years ago, complains of SOB. CXR was performed to assess for pulmonary oedema. Recent mammography was normal.

**i.** What are the differential diagnoses for the abnormality on the CXR (72a)?

**ii.** Given the features on CT (72b), is this a true or false aneurysm?

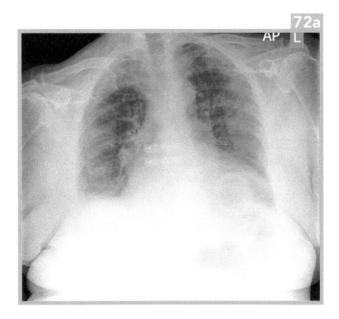

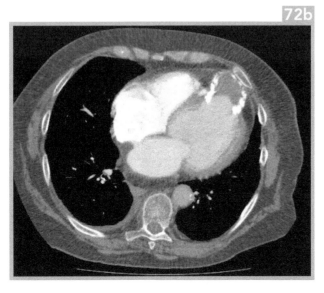

## Answer 72

**72i.** The CXR (72a) demonstrates a rim calcified 5 cm lesion overlying the left lower zone. The differential diagnoses for cystic structures in this position are breast cyst, bronchogenic cyst, pulmonary sequestration, pericardial cyst and LV aneurysm. Of all of these, the most likely to calcify to such an extent is the LV aneurysm.

**ii.** This is a true aneurysm. Figure 72b shows the aneurysm to be full of thrombus.

The two types of LV aneurysm are true and false. The true aneurysm is a bulging of the myocardium, usually at the site of an infarct. It may only be apparent in systole, where the characteristic paradoxical LV wall motion occurs and this is known as a functional LV true aneurysm.

A false aneurysm is not covered with myocardium (i.e. represents a myocardial rupture) and is only contained by fascia, usually pericardium. Classically, false aneurysms have a small neck and are limited only by adhesions within the pericardium. Thrombi are often found within the aneurysm and have a lamellated appearance on TTE, which can be misinterpreted as normal myocardial wall. The key feature is the paradoxical motion during the cardiac cycle. CT and MRI demonstrate thrombi exquisitely in cases where there is uncertainty. The main differential for intracardiac masses is intracardiac tumours, which can be demonstrated to show contrast enhancement on both CT and MRI. MRI can give further tissue characteristics of tumours and demonstrate late gadolinium enhancement in patients with LV infarction and paradoxical motion.

## QUESTION 73

73 A 59-year-old smoker with a previous anterior apical myocardial infarction presents to hospital with symptoms of left-sided hemiparesis. He is also known to have moderate left ventricular systolic dysfunction. He had a CT scan of his brain on this admission which confirmed that he had suffered an acute ischaemic stroke. His 12-lead ECG confirmed that he was in atrial fibrillation. As part of his routine stroke investigation, he had a transthoracic echocardiogram.

i.    What does Figure 73a show?

ii.   What does Figure 73b show?

iii.  What are the clinical uses of left ventricular opacification contrast?

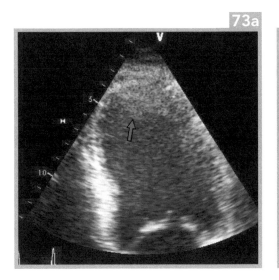

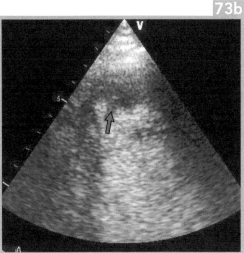

## Answer 73

**73i.** Figure 73a is a close-up view of the LV in the apical four-chamber view. There is a suspicion of a mass (arrow) attached to the thinned left ventricular apex. Given the clinical history, this may represent a left ventricular thrombus.

**ii.** To confirm the presence of an actual mass in the apical region and not just an artefact, left ventricular opacification contrast (Sonovue) was administered intravenously. Figure 73b shows the appearance following contrast administration. The left ventricular cavity appears white due to the presence of the contrast agent within the blood pool. The mass (arrow) is still evident confirming that the appearance on Figure 73a is not simply artefactual. Contrast echocardiography using agents such as Sonovue enhances the discrimination between myocardial tissue and the blood pool, by opacifying the left ventricular cavity while also making the myocardium appear darker. Left ventricular opacification is achieved by intravenous administration of microbubbles that consist of a gas contained by an outer shell. Sonovue consists of sulphur hexafluoride microbubbles with a phospholipid shell. The sulphur hexafluoride gas is exhaled through the lungs while the phospholipid component of the shell is metabolised by the body.

**iii.** In patients with suboptimal quality images, the use of left ventricular opacification contrast allows the echocardiographic diagnosis of apical thrombus, apical hypertrophic cardiomyopathy, ventricular noncompaction and ventricular pseudoaneurysm. It also allows improved endocardial visualisation for measurement of left ventricular volumes and ejection fraction. Left ventricular opacification contrast is also indicated for use in stress echocardiography when the endocardial definition of the LV is suboptimal (two or more contiguous endocardial segments).

# QUESTION 74

74  A 35-year-old male presents with a 3-month history of cough and some weight loss and was therefore referred by his GP for further investigation to exclude an underlying bronchogenic carcinoma.

i.   What does the CT demonstrate (74a–c)?

ii.  When would this structure normally disappear?

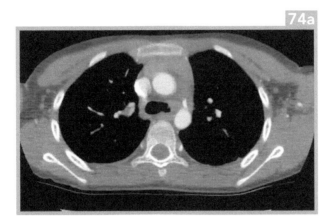

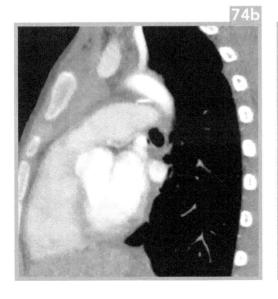

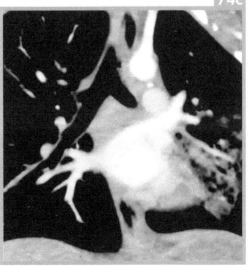

147

## Answer 74

**74i.** The CT images demonstrate a small PDA. The PDA connects the left pulmonary artery with the descending aorta beyond the origin of the left subclavian artery. Infective consolidation is seen in the left lower lobe in Figure 74c, consistent with a focal pneumonia.

**ii.** A PDA is associated with premature birth, birth asphyxia, rubella syndrome, coarctation, VSD and trisomy 18 and 20. Normally the ductus arteriosus functionally closes due to muscular contraction within 48 hours of birth, with 90% anatomically closing due to fibrosis and thrombosis by 2 months. Usually they are asymptomatic; however, the PDA can result in a shunt from the aorta to the pulmonary artery, into the lungs and then back to the left side of the heart. This can lead to an enlarged ascending aorta and arch; dilatation of the pulmonary vasculature; left atrial and left ventricular enlargement; and rarely, leads to congestive cardiac failure.

Treatment is either by medical means (antiprostaglandins) or surgical ligation.

# QUESTION 75

75  A 78-year-old female presents to the general cardiology clinic with a 6-month history of progressive breathlessness. Her GP had noted a loud murmur over her right parasternal area. She has no history of ischaemic heart disease or any significant past medical history. She is a nonsmoker. On auscultation, she had an ejection systolic murmur heard loudest at the upper right sternal border and no signs of heart failure. She was referred for a transthoracic echocardiography.

i.    What does the echocardiographic image show (75a)?

ii.   What is the natural history of this valvular disease?

iii.  If this patient had asymptomatic but severe disease, what other tests would be useful in guiding timing for surgery?

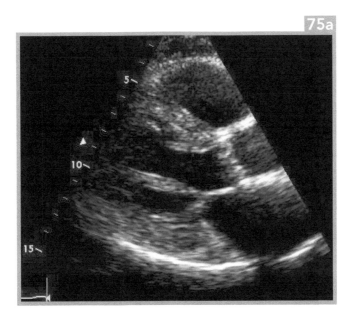

## Answer 75

**75i.** Figure 75b, acquired in the parasternal long-axis view, shows a calcified aortic valve (arrow) with the leaflets not in the 'open' position as would be expected during ventricular systole. Normal aortic valve opening in systole is shown in Figure 75c for comparison. There is left ventricular hypertrophy which is an adaptive response in aortic stenosis. The peak gradient across the valve is measured at 117 mmHg, with a mean gradient of 73 mmHg (75d). The calculated AVA by the continuity equation is 0.54 cm², as shown in Figure 75e. The echocardiographic definitions of severe aortic stenosis are: AVA ≤1 cm², peak pressure gradient ≥64 mmHg and mean pressure gradient ≥40 mmHg.

**ii.** An estimated 3–5% of the population above the age of 65 years has some degree of calcific degenerative aortic stenosis. Most of these patients are asymptomatic until the disease progresses to cause moderate-to-severe stenosis which often takes years, if not decades. The probability of remaining symptom-free with severe aortic stenosis without surgery is 82%, 67%, and 33% at 1, 2, and 5 years, respectively. When symptoms start to develop in severe aortic stenosis, the prognosis is poor in the absence of intervention, with survival rates of 30–50% at 5 years. The development of symptoms in severe aortic stenosis is a Class I indication for aortic valve replacement.

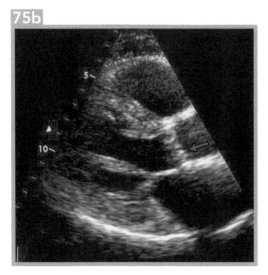

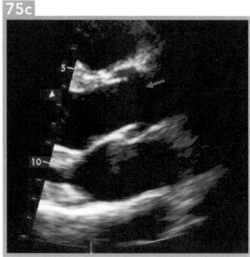

iii. Exercise stress echocardiography can provide prognostic information and helps risk stratify asymptomatic patients with severe aortic stenosis by assessing the increase in mean gradient across the aortic valve and the change in left ventricular systolic function with exercise. Exercise tolerance test is very useful in unmasking symptoms in patients who are apparently asymptomatic. It is safe to be undertaken in asymptomatic patients and should be a physician-supervised test. Parameters to monitor are the presence of symptoms, blood pressure response and ECG changes.

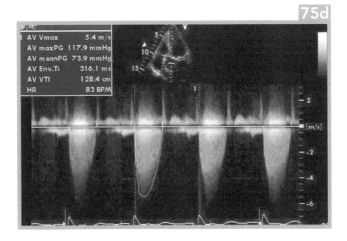

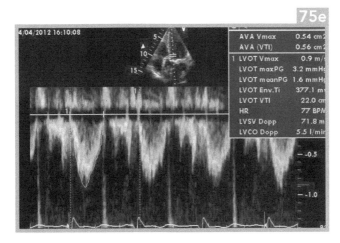

# INDEX

T - #0916 - 101024 - C160 - 246/174/7 - PB - 9781482235739 - Gloss Lamination